# Hockey For Parents

Mark James

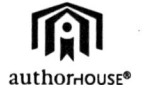

*AuthorHouse*™
*1663 Liberty Drive*
*Bloomington, IN 47403*
*www.authorhouse.com*
*Phone: 1-800-839-8640*

*© 2009 Mark James. All rights reserved.*

*No part of this book may be reproduced, stored in a retrieval system, or transmitted by any means without the written permission of the author.*

*First published by AuthorHouse 10/12/2009*

*ISBN: 978-1-4490-2954-8 (sc)*

*Printed in the United States of America*
*Bloomington, Indiana*

*This book is printed on acid-free paper.*

# About the Book

A review of hockey parents indicates an increasing number of parents who have not grown up with the game or have not played as children. The goal of this book was to create a simple hockey reference book targeted to these hockey parents, to better inform them of the strategies and basics of playing hockey. Parents offering instructions to their children, with the best of intentions, without a basic understanding of the fundamentals of the game, may be leading our young players astray. Hockey is a game of structure similar to chess. It requires the players to understand the basic systems of the game, and then to read and react to the opponents' moves. Thinking ahead and interpreting the play can only be developed with a strong understanding of the game. As a lot of parents get involved with hockey to volunteer and to be with their children, I decided to write a book to aid this understanding and to act as a handy reference. For the parents who have questions and are uncomfortable asking them, this book will hopefully answer some of the basic questions that come to mind when the whistle blows and the shouting from the stands begins. Parents, I believe, should develop knowledge of the game comparable to that of their child. This, in turn, will promote meaningful conversations which will lead to your child's improvement and success on the ice.

To new and experienced coaches there are sections in this book that will hopefully reinforce your training and act as basic reference material for the parents of your players as you lead your hockey team to success. These same basic principles have been employed from House League to "AAA" (traveling team) levels, all with success. The key is to measure player success on a player by player basis. Your evaluation, as coach, of the potential and ability of each player is critical when establishing your teaching plan. What may be a success for one player may be a disappointing result for another player. The weaker players, given realistic goals and achieving their goals, should be praised with full credit given. The stronger players relying on skill alone to score two goals a game, without passing and playing as a team player, will not achieve their full potential in a team environment. This selfish play may satisfy some parents who want to see their child score and carry the puck, but this type of player will soon fall from elite player status, and may even be dropped from the team with the parents wondering what went wrong.

Hockey is a game, but it is mainly a life lesson. Such a small percentage (way less than 1%) will ever make a living from hockey, so the focus must be on having fun and developing the skills necessary to succeed in the world. A growing number of coaches are insisting that good school marks be maintained or hockey will be the sacrificed. As most young players have a passion to play and to be with their friends, any chance of losing this opportunity is a strong motivator. I have found that positive hockey experiences, even with a lot of time away from the home, have led to improved marks for the players. They are forced to organize their time, complete assignments in advance, and with better physical health, are more alert. Major corporations put a strong emphasis, after education requirements, on hiring applicants who have achieved success in sports. These applicants understand teamwork (communication), time management, dedication and the sacrifice necessary to succeed. They bring this approach to their workplace.

Hockey can be fun for all, if played in a structured, well run and disciplined environment, with equal opportunity for all participants. A priority must be respect for all participants, including the referees. You, the parents in the stands, are the examples your children look up to. Don't take this responsibility lightly, as you are establishing the framework in which your child interacts with others. Unstructured environments are generally fun for the elite, but rarely fun for all. A well run team with clear rules is a successful and enjoyable team. Although winning is never the only goal, this type of team, when the pressure heats up, often finds a way to win. This puts the icing on the cake for a great and memorable experience.

To all the parents who have not played the game, or have played at the local level only, there is no shame in asking questions and learning from the coaches and other parents with experience. I relate this story of two friends. One is a businessman and the other is a self employed handyman and avid fisherman. The handyman invited the businessman and his kids out to fish one day, and as the hooks were baited some simple instructions were given to the kids by the handyman. The businessman listened, and continued to reinforce the instructions identically to his kids without question or resistance. The handyman was completely surprised that the businessman would accept the role of fisherman's assistant so easily and without resistance. When this was noted by the handyman, the response from the businessman was simple and logical, "You are the expert fisherman with many years of experience. Why would I not listen and heed your advice?" The point, often missed by most of us, is that you can learn from everybody and that most people have their own areas of expertise. You have to know when to park your ego at the door. If hockey is not your specialty (and playing house league or university recreation hockey does not make you an expert) then take advantage of the coach's experience, and that of any other parent with experience. This method will supply some honest and useful feedback that can only help in your child's development.

The head coach should also take advantage of the knowledge brought to the team by their assistants. You asked your assistant coaches for help; so listen to them and utilize them. Give them a definite role as in any business, and hold them accountable. Don't try to run the bench or practices as a one person show with assistants standing around or just collecting pucks. This rarely works, and does nothing to develop your staff and create teamwork. A team with 5 coaches, all teaching from the same playbook, will give the players more one on one time and better quality instruction.

Parents, please remember that you watch your child more closely than any coach or other parent, and you are bound to see more good than bad. I have seen parents walking out of the rink beaming that their child had played a superb game because their child had scored 2 or 3 goals. They are blissfully unaware that their child had missed two glorious chances to pass to a teammate for an easy goal. This same child had also been on the ice for four goals against the team, and was responsible for making bad defensive mistakes, completely ignoring the team's defensive strategies developed in practice. Parents, the point is to seek out feedback, and to be willing to listen and share that feedback with your child.

If you are a parent with legitimate experience, then please try this. Pick out one of the **non** top 6 players. After a strong game, by that child's standards, point out the strong points and shake the player's hand. You have just made that player's day, and reinforced the value of that player's play to the team. Without all the players improving and contributing, the team will never achieve its goals. The old adage "you are only as strong as your weakest link" is just as true on a hockey team as in life.

# Dedication

I would like to take this opportunity to thank the people I love, as it can never be said enough times how much their support and patience means. It has been said many times that "behind every man is a great woman" and in my case no truer words could be uttered. Nancy has stood constantly by my side through the good and the bad times and without her management of our family and especially me, nothing would ever get done. I was blessed with 4 boys (Michael, Matthew, Markus and Mackenzie) who have all played or continue to play the game we love called Hockey. They have endured my coaching, my parenting, and my constant insistence that they perform to the best of their abilities. They have been taught to measure their success by being able to leave whatever activity they attempt with their heads held high, knowing they have given their mental and physical best. Making the NHL, for us, has never been the measure of success. The adult you become as a result of the lessons learned from this marvelous game is that measure. As parents, Nancy and I could not be more proud.

To my parents, Ron and Jan, who came to Canada from England after the Second World War, I would like to offer my gratitude. They dedicated a major part of their young lives to driving me and my sister Corinne (a successful figure skater) all over North America at great expense and personal sacrifice. They became new hockey parents with no background or experience with the game. They worked around one car, trying to support a family on long hours and one income that inevitably led to many missed or late dinners that went unmentioned. I can never say thank you enough. Two stories will stick with me forever and I would like to share them with you as a fellow hockey parent. Both my parents could not ice skate upon arriving in Canada. Although they eventually owned skates, they never became comfortable skating and avoided it at all costs. When I was a young player, father/son hockey games were the norm. Most of the fathers had played hockey and therefore could skate at least sufficiently enough to compete against 7 or 8 years olds. In order to not let me down my dad strapped on the skates and gave it a go. I remember clearly my dad holding onto the boards for dear life, trying not to fall and crack his coconut, while the game proceeded around him with the occasional pass from another parent to try and keep him involved. I wondered at the time why could my father not be like the other fathers. It took many years to realize the unbelievable courage and support that my dad gave me that day. He put my feelings ahead of his; absorbing the obvious discomfort and embarrassment he must have felt that day. We will talk about team and supporting your teammates a lot in this book but you have to be willing to sacrifice your personal feelings at all cost to help your teammates. That is the true sign of courage and team. Dad, you taught me that, and if it hasn't been said enough, thank you.

My mom took on the roll of hockey instructor, and taught me to shoot a puck out back of our apartment building. My mom was always there for me and remained supportive throughout my hockey career. As I moved on to University Hockey my parents continued to drive great distances to watch my games. I remember in university when the drinking age was 19 and I had hardly turned 18 (I was the youngest on the team). I was playing with many guys well into their 20's and my parents still attended my games. After a game in those days, the next place of business to celebrate a win or a loss was the local bar. My teammates were great, and seeing my parents there, introduced themselves and said "Come on Ron and Jan, we are going for a drink. You're welcome to join us". To my chagrin, my parents accepted. I remember to this day my mother looking at my face and reading my discomfort; partly as I was underage and my parents were strict; partly as I was the youngest and no one else's parents were there, let alone joining us for a drink. My mom pulled me aside and gave me a quick life lesson all parents should relate to, as your time is coming. My mom looked me straight in the eye and said, "Mark we have driven you to almost every rink around. We only have our closest friends left. Our other friends are all gone as we were never available to see them as we were always at your hockey. We come to your games, as we have for the last 15 years, as we have nowhere else to go and we enjoy watching your hockey." I realized once again that if it wasn't for their effort and sacrifice I would not have had the opportunities I had then and have today.

We then went for that drink. Mom, many thanks, I hope I paid.

I have been lucky to have great in-laws in Bill and Bunny who have played a large role in the growth of our boys off the ice, and in supporting their daughter without falter. Their support of me is also greatly appreciated, with Bunny spending many hours as the invaluable editor of this book. With the rapid growth of hockey in North America for young ladies, I wanted to ensure the book was gender neutral. I therefore used the plural term "their" in many instances where "him" or "her" were grammatically correct. For this I accept responsibility. I put it down to author's prerogative and should not reflect on the excellent work of the editor.

I have been blessed with a large family (holidays at our house has been known to be busy) and since this may be my only book, I would like to acknowledge you individually. My sister Corinne, Joe and their girls Rachel and Sophie, Brother-in-law Les, Cheryl, son Scott (Holly and their daughters Averie and Addison), daughter Janine, Brother-in-law John, Shelley, son Brayden (our fifth son), Brother-in-law Doug, Joey, son Sam and daughter Kaliegh, Sister-in-law Wendy, Ron, son Billy, daughters Jenny (Mark daughters Breyena and Madison), Krista and Nicole. To brother in-law Steve and Grandparents, you are greatly missed.

# Table of Contents

| <u>**Chapters**</u> | <u>**Page #**</u> |
|---|---|
| 1. Team Rules – The Basics | 1 |
| 2. The Basic Principles (BP) | 6 |
| 3. The Pre Game Talk, After Game Review and Team Play Book | 11 |
| 4. The Dump-In Versus Carrying the Puck In. | 22 |
| 5. The Powerplay Offensive End | 26 |
| 6. The Power Play Breakout | 30 |
| 7. The Penalty Kill Fore-check | 32 |
| 8. The Penalty Kill Box in Our End | 37 |
| 9. 5 Player Fore-check | 43 |
| 10. 5 Player Defensive Positioning in Our End (the centerman's role) | 47 |
| 11. Face-offs in the Defensive End | 52 |
| 12. Face-offs in the Offensive End | 61 |
| 13. How to Correctly Execute a 2 on 1 | 65 |
| 14. How To Correctly Execute a 3 on 2 | 68 |

15. Playing Defense.
   The Toughest Job in Hockey. ... 71
16. Body Checking and Angling ... 86
17. Changing Lines -
   when to change and when not to. ... 89
18. Close the Gap ... 96
19. The Lights Out Drill-- Knowing where
   all 12 players are at all times. ... 100
20. Acceptable Behavior from the Parents. ... 104
21. Pulling the Goalie ... 119
22. Dropped Your Stick? Then Pick it Up! ... 123
23. Why Do Officials Keep Blowing
   Their Whistles? ... 126
24. Penalties and How To Deal with
   Multiple Calls on the Same Play ... 137
25. What is the Penalty Call Sign Language? ... 146
26. The Game and Book is Over –
   How to Contact Us. ... 153
27. Glossary ... 155
28. Penalty Suspensions ... 159

# 1
# TEAM RULES – THE BASICS

*Don't make a rule you are not willing to enforce.*

Teams should establish rules and make them effective for all, despite the consequences. These rules must be fully adhered to by all bench and support staff. Every team rule is set in place for a reason, and must be fully supported by the parents. Rules that require kids and coaches to be at the arena at a certain time must be enforced, and penalties must be administered if rules are not followed. Most of us start work every day at a set time, and consistent lateness is not accepted. Being late does nothing to promote you within any organization. Coaches, **don't make a rule you are not going to enforce.** Parents must fully support the rules of the team, and therefore should make time at the beginning of the season to review the rules and state their concerns. If you have a certain situation, such as potential lateness on certain days, and it is contrary to one of the rules, then make it known in the parent meeting, and get concurrence as to what you will commit to. Any non conformance to team rules should be an extreme exception and because you work late is not a sufficient excuse. In the case of lateness, parents should make other driving arrangements. If there are absolutely no other options, then work with the team on what you can commit to. We have all stood for that horrible hour before the game making idle chatter, and then, the one parent who is always late finally arrives- late again! You know the feeling you would have after rushing from your work or responsibilities to fulfill your commitment, only to see the player who has arrived late start the game without penalty. Penalties should be for repeat offenses, and not for bad weather and other emergencies, as safety must be given first priority. Parents should plan to leave early enough and to avoid lateness issues.

Good parents will take the lead, and ensure that the rules are enforced, even away from the ice. I use the example that if the coach has asked to be called "Coach Mark", then when having discussions at home use, "Coach Mark" not "Mark". If you say something like, "Go ask Mark," you are making it difficult for the child to adjust when they do approach the coach. No player or parent is above the rules. Every effort should be made to adjust your rules or preferences at home to accommodate team rules. Some basic rules that should be discussed in every team's opening meeting would include;

1. Set the time at which every member of the team is required to be at the rink for games and practices.

2. Establish the acceptable dress requirement for all members of the team. As much as it looks nice when everyone is in matching track suit, leather jacket, hat etc., this is already an expensive sport

without forcing additional cost. If someone is willing to sponsor the clothing, then that is terrific. Otherwise, a black pair of pants and white shirt or turtleneck should be quite acceptable.

3. No swearing, racial comments, taunting, or bullying, will be tolerated at any time.

4. Respect for teammates, coaching staff, opposing team, and coaches and referees is expected at all times. Parents should be willing to support the coaches to increase game suspension above league rules for repeated offenses. For situations where a penalty was not called on the ice but the coach observed unacceptable behaviour by a player, then team discipline may be taken by the coaching staff and requires the support of the parents.

5. Continuing with respect, I am a firm believer, especially at the younger levels (as noted above), that the coaching staff should be referred to as Coach (first name of coach), or Mr. (last name of coach). A six year old shouting across the dressing room, "Hey Mark, pass me my stick," should receive zero response until the request is changed to, "Coach Mark, could you pass me my stick **please?**" Basic manners, such as the use of please and thank you, still go a long way.

6. Respect again. Parents' conduct will affect your child's playing time. If you yell and swear at the referee your child's playing time will most likely be reduced: be ejected from the arena, and some

associations rules force the coaching staff to identify the player whose relative was ejected, and that player is removed from the game. If you want to embarrass yourself, and especially your child, in front of teammates and friends, this is an easy way to do it.

7. All medical information, plus any information requested by the trainers to do their job properly, must be completed and submitted at the commencement of the season. All injuries must be reported to the trainer even if they do not occur on the ice.

8. All players should have their own water bottles.

9. No horseplay in the arena or the dressing room. You are representing your team and center at all times. Throwing of ice from your skates, tossing tape or any other object should not be tolerated.

10. Managing is a difficult enough job, and I hold the greatest respect for the people who volunteer for this very time consuming and demanding role. We, as parents, must do everything possible to make their task easier. If you get an e-mail, respond with a confirmation every time, even if you don't have the answer to the request at that time. Schedules and changes should be published as far in advance as possible to allow for proper planning and car pooling if required.

11. Parents and players are responsible, not the Coaching Staff, for ensuring their equipment is safe and meets all standards. Parents must ensure that sticks are taped, skates are sharpened, and everything necessary to play is packed and brought to the arena. Team trainers should carry extra helmet screws and clips and maybe an extra neck guard and mouth guard in original packaging. If the new mouth guard is used, the player now owns it, and must replace it with a new similar guard prior to the next practice or game.

Keep the list short and simple. Parents, remember that the beginning of the year is the time to discuss and agree on the rules, not when the rules are in question.

# 2

# THE BASIC PRINCIPLES (BP)

*Constant Motion*
*Maintain eye contact on the puck at all times.*
*Create Space on the ice.*
*Create odd man advantages.*
*Defend by being closer to your net*
*than the player you are covering.*
*The puck moves faster than the player -*
*utilize the pass.*
*Control the puck.*
*Communicate to teammates at all times.*
*Hockey is a Team Sport.*
*When on defense think offense -*
*when on offense think defense.*

Throughout this book we will always come back to the fact that every play, concept and approach to hockey should be geared to meet the basic principles noted below. Every game has a focus, and every drill and lesson should always be based on the basic principles of hockey.

1. **<u>Hockey is a speed sport with constant motion</u>**. Success is achieved by the best physically and mentally conditioned teams out-playing their opponents. This can only be done by keeping your feet in constant motion. One example of lack of

motion occurs when wingers come into their zone and stop on the hash marks. This is taught by a lot of coaches, but hockey is not place to place. Stay in motion by coming in parallel to the boards about the face-off dot away from the boards, pivoting, always facing the play, and accelerating up the boards, or breaking to an opening. There are times when a defenseman must fire a puck around the boards in an emergency situation, and the winger must go to the boards and ensure that the puck is trapped or tipped out of the zone. This is a critical part of the game, where motion must be sacrificed to make the play. The key is that no play should start with a winger stopping on purpose. Another example may be an offensive player standing motionless in front of the other team's goalie. Stay in motion, coming in and out of the area around the net, and put pressure on the defender to watch you and the puck simultaneously. Lastly, the easiest target for an opponent to hit is one standing still. Staying in motion allows you the ability to avoid a body check. Don't slow to pass, shoot, and then remain on a straight path to admire it. This will lead to one easy target to hit. YOU!

2. **<u>Maintain eye contact with the puck at all times.</u>** Put your body in a position to simultaneously see the puck and the player you are defending, or the net you are trying to score into. As a general principle, all turns should be made with the player facing the play at all times. You can't keep your

eye on the puck if you aren't facing the play. For this reason, all players are taught to stop and turn in both directions. Turning your back on the puck should only be done in extreme emergencies, and in most defensive emergencies, facing the puck and cutting off the pass is still the best possibility of recovery.

3. **<u>Create space</u>**. The ice surface is a large playing area, utilize it all. Remember that the puck moves faster than any player, and offensive players make better decisions when they have more time to get their heads up and think. Defending players therefore are taught to keep close to the offensive players and take space away at all times, thus forcing the offensive player into quick, rushed decisions. These rushed decisions are usually not the best executed decisions. Wayne Gretzky made a living behind the opponent's net. This area was a lightly guarded area, and gave him the most time to read the play and make the appropriate decision.

4. **<u>Create odd man opportunities</u>** such as 3 on 2's, 2 on 1's. Do this by utilizing quick puck movement. A triangle type offense used correctly, with maximum size to the triangle, is the cornerstone to all play. A scrum on the boards will be won, the majority of the time, by the team with the most players in the scrum. In simple terms, do whatever is possible to have more players in the play than the other team.

5. **<u>When defending put yourself closer to your own goal than the player you are covering.</u>** The best position would be directly between the player and your goalie. Keep the puck and player you are covering away from your goal, and you are in the right position.

6. The **<u>puck moves faster than you can skate</u>** so head man the puck, but don't force the pass for the sake of passing. Passing at the right time is the key to hockey.

7. **<u>Maintain control of the puck</u>**. If we have the puck, they can't score. A basic example of control involves not throwing the puck around the boards when a direct pass to the stick is an option. Don't dump the puck in if you can gain the blue line with the puck under control. Bring the puck back toward your own end (defense to defense) and start again under control if necessary, but don't just dump it back off the boards in an effort to go forward.

8. **<u>Constant verbal communication</u>** amongst players is critical to strong team play. Examples in your own end may include; helping find the open man, telling a teammate they have pressure ("Man on") identifying your defensive zone coverage assignments, entering the zone. Examples in the offensive zone may include; who is going to the net and who is the high player in the slot. Talking on the bench in between shifts is important and should

be encouraged for strong team communication. Players cannot communicate too much.

9. **<u>Hockey is a Team sport</u>** and the success of the team has to be put 100% above the success of the player. I personally hate individual awards, and I avoid reading game sheets and showing season point stats to young players. I especially would advise all parents against paying for goals. If you want to pay for anything, pay your child for every plus (goals for your team, less goals against, while that player is on the ice- excluding power plays and penalty kills). If your child is constantly plus, the team will be successful.

10. **<u>When on defense think offense, and when on offense think defense.</u>** The best players in the world have the ability to read and react, but each player must anticipate a turnover. They must make sure they are positioning themselves to take advantage of a turnover for a quick break, or be in a defensive position (third player high) to quickly get back on defense on a lost turnover.

# 3

# THE PRE GAME TALK, AFTER GAME REVIEW AND TEAM PLAY BOOK

*Mental preparation is as important as the physical preparation*

Parents spend all kinds of money each year arranging for extra ice time to improve their kids' skating, shooting and stick handling. They often ignore the mental part of the game which many believe is the most important part of hockey. All the power skating and skills schools are necessary and vital to the growth of the hockey player, but where is the focus on the mental part of the game? Sure it is easy to drop your kid off at camp and watch, if you want to see someone skate your child to exhaustion and run them through drills. However, very few camps ever take the time to show the players why they are learning the skills, how they are used in a game, and how the skills are effective when reading and reacting to different situations. The reason is simple. It is very difficult to simulate game situations and utilize ice time for 20 kids to ensure that each child understands mentally what is required. So most schools take the easy way out and treat everyone equally. They run the drills, get a sweat on the players and send them back to Mommy and Daddy. Parents rarely receive a written document explaining what was taught during the course and/or the reasons for those lessons. This makes it difficult for anyone to make sure the knowledge is retained by the player. Within two weeks players are back to their old habits as current coaches didn't see the skills taught. They have nothing to review in writing about why the skills were taught, and therefore they don't reinforce those skills. While any extra ice time is good, the results could be further maximized with proper reference material. This material can be retained and shared with the coach and player at a later date, making everyone aware of what was taught in the course.

Parents must insist that part of the hockey curriculum include at least 40% off ice instruction on the basics of the game, the reason for performing the skills, and what is expected once you hit the ice. This can be accomplished by separate meetings, or by utilizing time a half hour before hitting the ice. Using time after practice doesn't seem to work as well for this purpose, as the kids are tired and the parents want to go home. Perhaps more importantly, the player has to remember what was said for days before they get a chance to try it. Establish separate days during the month to go to a gym, parking lot or outdoor arena. Walk through power plays, penalty kills and all areas of the game, with a ball and whistle. Have the kids stop in place and discuss positional errors, pointing out corrections. Why waste valuable and expensive ice time to teach the basics, when the hour on ice can be spent in full motion working on what was learned in the gym. Some coaches will even establish their standard drills, assign them a name, and then, when on the ice will call out a drill by name. The players will break to their respective places on the ice, and the drill commences, saving valuable time. It is also easy to plan a practice for assistant coaches when they are told the 5 drill names in the order they will be run. They can then have cones, pucks, and whatever else is needed, ready to go while the current drill is running. Parents must work with their child to ensure that they fully understand the names of the drills and the drill requirements. Parents should also attend these off-ice sessions, and learn, along with their kids, so that meaningful conversation or clarification of areas being taught can be discussed at a later time.

This 40% mental teaching can also be in the 10 minutes before going on the ice. This is a good time to refresh the strategies and reinforce the latest practice teachings. A brief three to five minutes after the game can also be used to recap the successes and review any weak areas identified. These weaknesses would be natural topics for next practices. My opening speech to parents and players every year is, "If this team is the best prepared and smartest team by the start of playoffs, we will have a chance at winning the championship." The players and parents must believe in the "System." This is my term, but in my opinion every team needs to hang their team goals on the back of some identifiable slogan. All players, coaches, and parents should be able to relate to, and state, the basics of the "System." The "System" contains the fundamental rules of the team. If these are followed by the players, while working together as a team, this will lead to team success. The coaches and parents must continually emphasize the successes that result from using the fundamentals of the "System." They must also highlight examples of breakdowns that could have been avoided by proper implementation of the "System." Reinforcement can occur before, during, or after the game, until complete buy-in is embraced by all.

So, how do you know a "System" is being bought into by the players? What, as a parent, do you look for? I like to break coaching involvement into stages as follows. These stages are necessary, and have been proven over a period of many years of coaching. It is critical that the parents understand the process for implementing the "System," and are fully supportive, publicly and at home. If you have questions, approach the coach for clarification. (BP "communicate")

**<u>Stage 1.</u>** This is the initial introduction of expectations, and should occur in the first month of the season. Team rules, expectations, and parts of the "System" are explained and taught during this time. This is a strict stage where conflict may occur between players and coaches. The players are asked to follow the system 100% in order to give the "System" a chance to help the team improve. This is a difficult stage as players generally grasp the concepts at different paces. It is also a difficult time for the players as all their past experiences and teachings may not be identical to the current team plan. Creative players are capable of finding success outside of the system, and may potentially challenge any "System" if it is a new approach. These players need to be encouraged to stay within the "System," playing as a team member, and helping their line mates and teammates with proper positioning and play. **Coaches need to be highly vocal, positively reinforcing on-ice players to assist with reading the play, and recommending proper reactions to that read of the play. Focus of coaches should be on getting players into the correct positions per the "System," and giving the players the best opportunity to succeed.**

<u>**Stage 2.**</u> The key part, in this stage, is execution and willingness to fail while trying it. No player should be criticized for trying to follow the "System." The players' ability to read the play, and their reactions, are not trained to game speed, and therefore they will often make the wrong decision. For safety reasons, in the early years of a player's development, players are instructed to move the puck around the boards to a winger at the hash marks in their own end. As the players develop to the next stage, the defense will be asked to carry the puck out of the zone more often. What can happen, as the player learns to read the game situation, is that the defenseman will see the winger covered on the boards, and will try to carry the puck as the coach has instructed. The defenseman makes an easy mistake of not seeing an opposing player coming towards them and is stripped of the puck resulting in a goal against. At this time, I have seen too many coaches get upset with the player, so that the player, for the rest of the game, throws the puck safely along the

boards to a covered winger rather than make a mistake rushing the puck.  So in this example, confidence is shot, and progress stops.  A tip for parents and coaches is to ask the player what they saw, and why they made the read that they did.  Find the positive from what the player tells you, and try to give instructional points to improve the player's ability to read the play.  This will allow the player to better react to that situation in the future.  In this case, knowing where all players are on the ice at all times is the key to making the right read.  If the play is not there, maybe reversing the play, or simply just getting it out of the zone until our abilities grow, is the best alternative.  **Coaches should be moderately vocal (positively) at this point, but can now be more selective; aiding the puck carrier with their reading of the play but focusing more on the players who are not in control of the puck.**

**Stage 3.** This is a stage when the players are grasping the "System" and the coaches' expectations. The players will start to ask questions of the coaching staff. Communication at this stage is direct to the coaches, and may prompt questions such as, "Can we do this within the "System?", "If I read this, can I do this, or throw this kind of pass?". This is a very positive stage, and all players come into this stage by the second month but at various times and intensity. Always first ask the player what they are thinking, and how their question ties to the "System" in their opinion. The basic rules and "System" don't change, but we are developing and expanding their experience as players, and how they react within the basic principles of the "System." Examples of game situations influencing the "System" are 1) our team will push on offense if we are down a goal late in the game-- or 2) play more conservatively with a third and maybe fourth player high in the other team's zone if we are up a goal. Players will learn to read the game situation and alter the team strategy in coordination with the coaching staff. **Coaches are becoming less vocal to on-ice players. They are spending more time answering questions, and using the mini arena whiteboards on the bench to point out positioning and key teaching points. Parents, if the team is not into Stage 3 by the end the second month of the season, it is time for the parents and coaching staff to meet and assess why this is not yet happening.**

<u>Stage 4.</u> My favorite stage, and the one I love seeing, is the reaction of the bench staff as they have watched the progress from Stage 1. They probably felt the push back earlier on from some of the players. However, the bench staff had agreed that all players would adopt the "System" and non conformance was not to be an option. Remember, rules are equal for all, with no exceptions. Stage 4 is when the players continue to communicate with their coaches but also start to communicate with each other. They come off the ice discussing the good and bad of their last shift and how they are going to make changes to improve the next shift. This is the most enjoyable stage, as the coaching staff moves into game management mode and away from the full-out teaching

mode.  It is also great to hear the communication, and to hear the positive self confidence brought out by the players.  They now know what is expected, and they are now working together to improve their situational game reads and reactions.   The players, from experience, don't even realize they have entered Stage 4 until asked how they found the game with the coaching staff so quiet.  Player confidence is growing quickly as the players realize that they are all on the same page.  Coaches are allowing the players to go play their game with minimal on-ice instruction.  Players are freed up to focus on their game, and should be finding success far beyond the start of the year. **At this stage the coaching staff will have seriously limited their need for on-ice instruction. The coaches are mostly focused on bench whiteboard instruction and game management.  Increased game management time may, for example, afford time for the coaching staff to gain tactical advantage by matching lines with the other team.  Practice time can now include working on set or trick plays that may come in useful late in the year or in the playoffs.**

<u>**Stage 5.**</u>  This is the final stage when the statement and commitment that "the smartest team by the end of the year will put you in a position to play for a championship" comes true.  It is at this time that you step back as a coach and the team drives itself to success.  The team believes in the "System" 100%, they believe in themselves 100%, and they believe they can succeed 100%.  The coaching staff is solely there for

game management and opening the door. The team is so comfortable with the expectations and requirements of the "System," so that as the pressure increases and competition mistakes occur, our team works the "System", remaining calm and focused. **Coaches at this stage are focused on game management and positive reinforcement after each shift.**

One year stands out as my favorite Stage 5 example. This occurred the first year I held the role of head coach (at the age of 16) for a young house league team. All the other coaches were fathers and experienced coaches. Our staff had no coaching experience, so we started with common sense, and drew from our personal playing experiences. Our teachings were the basics strategies of what later was pulled together and improved upon to be known as the "System." We started logically, with everyone being taught the basic skills of hockey and we progressed from there. We were very vocal in the early stages, and worked hard on the mental part of the game. We continued to get better as a team and made the play-offs, but not as the first place team. From all the championships and tournaments won, I can't remember coming first in the regular season. **The season is for developing all your players equally, not about winning.** We moved through the round robin portion of the playoffs even though we were still in Stage 3. Most players still were requiring positive vocal direction on the ice from the coaching staff. The mental preparation, the pre-game talks, the post game wrap ups, and the dedication to the "System" had taken us, surprisingly, to the Championship game. The parents, who had sat in the dressing rooms and attended practices, had played a big supporting role. They asked questions while understanding the "System," and were a big factor in helping teach their children in support of the coaching staff. Without the parents' support we would not have made it that far. The Championship pre-game meeting in the dressing room began with an eerie confidence despite the fact that the team we were playing had defeated us on previous occasions. The kids were asked to believe in the "System" as this had got us to the Championship game. More importantly, they were asked to relax and to just go have fun. The team had moved to the edge of Stage 4 late in the playoffs, and the coaching staff was all set to help the boys play the Championship game. I remember to this day all the excitement of that Championship game. Watching the first shift with my assistant coach (a fellow 16 year old) we fully expected to say something to the players on the ice to support and help them. The first shift was a complete surprise, as the players moved according to the "System" and had a positive shift. Buzzers were used in those days, and after the first 3 minutes, we looked at each other and realized we had offered no on-ice instruction for the entire shift. This was definitely a first. Pats on the helmets were given for all players as they came through the door. The second set of players went out, and then a third, and by the second period we had not uttered an on-ice instruction. We had the game firmly in hand. By the third period, we sat on the top of the bench and watched the players come off and go on the ice as though we were not there. A complete movement to Stage 5 had occurred, with utter success for every player on the team. A Championship was theirs! The smiles on the faces of every player and parent were clear indications of a fun and successful season.

# 4

# THE DUMP-IN VERSUS CARRYING THE PUCK IN.

*Use the dump-in to facilitate time to change players.*
*Dump the puck in away from the goalie.*
*The dump breaks down the trap.*

Almost all parents want to see their kid carry the puck into the defending zone, beat one or more defenders, and score the T.V. highlight goal. In reality this rarely happens. The basic rules for crossing the red line go directly to the basic principle (BP) that if you have an odd man advantage (2 on 1 or 3 on 2) then carry the puck and run the plays to be discussed in later chapters. If you are even at 3 on 3 or out numbered at 2 on 3, then take advantage of the situation and dump the puck into the zone. Fore-check the other team's defense to regain possession and gain the zone. Too many teams do not utilize this situation to execute a proper line change, and they turn the puck over trying to stickhandle, or make low percentage passes allowing the other team to counter attack. This quick counter attack puts major pressure on your own defense that may have needed a change, and needed the puck dumped deep to make that change. Too many times I see players who are at the end of a 1 minute shift attempting to carry the puck into the opposition's zone when they don't have an odd man advantage. The other team steals the puck, counterattacks, and traps the same players on the ice for another 30 to 40 seconds. Now the defending group is tired, and if the other team is properly coached they have made their player changes. This is the time when most defensive breakdowns occur, and goals against are scored. Overall, players must evaluate the situation as they near the red line. If it is not an odd man advantage then dump the puck in and change.

As a Read and React note – if the defense are backing into the zone and giving the offensive player room to gain the zone unimpeded, even if you are out numbered, take what is given and drive to the corner. This gives your teammates more time to change. Remember that you should never give the puck away if you don't have to.

The dump-in is a useful offensive tool, but too often an improper dump-in is completely ineffective and only serves to turn over the puck. When players are extremely tired and in need of a change, giving the puck away on a dump-in is a wise decision. A dump-in used to gain territory, not to give the puck away. Here are some key points to review with your child:

1. Never dump the puck in at the goalie. This is cute when the players are Novice because, once in a while, the puck may go in, or a large rebound occurs due to the inexperience of the goalie. This type of chance happens rarely as players get older. The goalie is more likely to take control of the puck

and cause a face off, or pass to an open teammate. Even a puck easily shot down the boards that goes behind the net allows experienced goalies to stop it and control it. This would also be an unnecessary turn over.

2. The correct dump-in is executed as you cross center ice. The forwards should be timing themselves to cross the blue line at full speed as the puck is shot across the blue line. The player dumping the puck must not force his forwards to hold up or delay at the blue line or the advantage is lost. The player dumping the puck with only one forward ahead of him should focus the dump-in into that corner away from the goalie. The most effective dump-ins are generally; a hard cross ice dump-in (figure A. A.), a soft dump-in to the close corner (figure A. B.), or a hard wrap around dump-in (figure A. C.).

3. The dump-in is a good offensive tool to move the puck up the ice, and to get into the offensive zone. In late parts of the game, when the other team is protecting a lead by playing the trap, (3 to 4 players all in the neutral area creating in effect a wall for the offense to try to break through), trying to stickhandle into the zone without losing control of the puck is risky. The dump will break through the wall, and get the puck deep where the team that wants it the most will recover it.

## The Dump-in Figure A

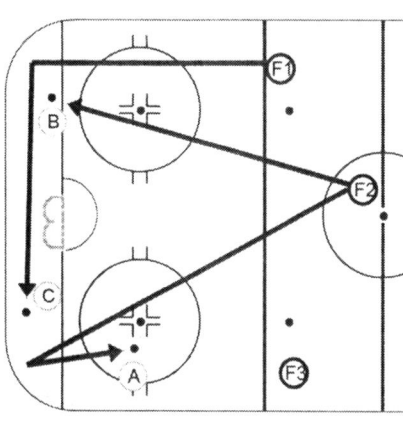

A. The hard cross-ice dump angled to bounce back toward the checking forward

B. The soft dump to the same side corner

C. The hard wrap around dump to the far winger for recovery

# 5

# THE POWERPLAY OFFENSIVE END

*Move the puck quickly and create space.*
*Create odd man advantages.*
*Players should constantly move*
*to break down the box.*
*Pressure into the box to force defensive coverage errors*
*Work for a shot from a quality scoring area.*
*2 or more players on the puck recovery*

Once you have gained the defensive zone, there are many options and ideas from different coaches on how to attack the defensive positions. Remember that the main goal is to move the puck around the exterior of the defensive box quickly, with lots of player movement. Players are trying to draw the defenders out of position, and to create openings to break down the box. On the power play (Figure B. Standard) the general positions to the right attacking side of the net are: the center below the goal line, the right winger on the hash marks and the left winger moving from high slot, to the front of net to wide left of the defensive box. Two players are against one defender giving the offense the advantage. It is then up to the offensive players to move the puck quickly and to break to open areas, causing the defenders to react and alter their coverage. This movement will hopefully force the defenders to make a mistake in their communications, leaving an offensive player open in a key shooting area.

The key to the power play is to break down the box, creating openings to move inside the box to key shooting locations. Anytime a defender is overly aggressive, stretching the box by charging out to the puck carrier, it opens up a simple give-and-go return pass opportunity into the area vacated by the defender. This can create a scoring opportunity.

The puck moved back to the defense allows the puck to switch sides of the ice rink, moving the defenders, and allowing the offensive team to try to break down the other side of the defenders. A shot is always a possibility, and is best when the offensive defenseman can move to the center of the ice (Figure B. Umbrella). This gives the offensive defenseman outlets to the left and right depending on which offensive forward attacks. If no one comes to the defenseman, leaving a shooting lane to the net, the player can shoot, and the bottom forwards should drive the net to screen or deflect the shot and put in any rebounds lying around.

Remember every coach has set plays, picks, or other items that they want their teams to perform, but the key to any successful power play is quick movement of the puck. Movement, and constant pressure into the box area by all the offensive players, puts pressure on the defenders to continue to move, and to look for their coverage assignments. This constant movement of the puck, and players cutting through the critical box area, is so important to forcing a defensive coverage mistake that will ultimately lead to success. Moving the puck around the outside of the defensive box serves a purpose if used to gain an advantageous position or scoring opportunity, but prolonged movement, more than 10 seconds outside the box, does nothing but waste time which is what the defense wants.

On a last note, puck recovery after a shot or a misdirected pass is the most critical part of the power play. At this time defenders can, by clearing the puck down the ice, waste 10 seconds or more and can get to the bench for a player change. Once you lose the puck on the man advantage, the power play team must immediately throw one more player than the opposition onto the puck to regain the puck. If the defenders have 2 then the offense must have three. A painful time watching youth hockey is seeing 2 forwards, after a shot is deflected into the corner, continuing to stand in front of the net. They proceed to yell at the third forward who is fighting 2 defenders for the puck. They are asking that player to pass them the puck so they can score and be the hero (and get $5 from their grandparent). This odd man advantage on the puck for the penalty killing team is unlikely to end up with the puck coming out to the 2 players awaiting the pass in front of the net. Players should get to the corner and recover the puck, making sure they have more players on the puck than the defending team. This may mean a defenseman must leave the point to help fight for the puck if necessary. If they don't do this, chances are they are going to skate all the way back to their end to set up and try again. The skate to the corner is closer.

# The Power Play Offensive End
## Figure B

### Power Play Offensive End - Standard

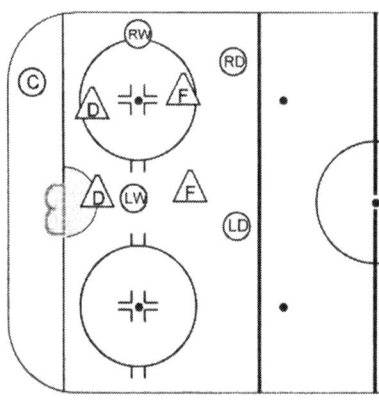

Standard positioning: with 3 players overloading one side, with center below the goal line, winger on the boards, and (RD) high at the point. Goal is to have 3 players move the puck outside of defensive box against 2 attackers thus having the player advantage on one side of the ice.

### Power Play Offensive End - Umbrella

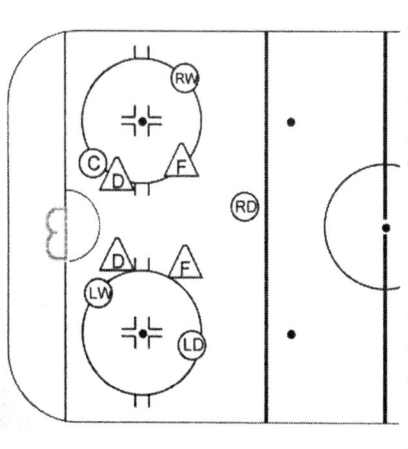

Positioning: (RD) gets to the middle of the ice near the blue line for the best shooting position and ability to go left or right with the pass. Goal is to draw one [F] to them and open up the side that [F] has vacated. Slow response to the (RD) by either [F] means a great opportunity to shoot, with (LW) and (C) to screen and collect a rebound.

# 6

# THE POWER PLAY BREAKOUT

*Control the puck in your end.*
*Set up behind the net to allow your team*
*to get into their positions.*
*Break out as a team with speed.*

The power play starts with a solid breakout, generally beginning with one of the defenseman stopping behind the net. This gives the other players time to get to their assigned area of the ice so that they can begin to move in unison up the ice. One of my pet peeves in minor hockey, is the practice of placing offensive players up near the defending team's blue line. In most cases I see offensive players standing still waiting for the breakout and then cutting across the ice trying to get a pass. This breaks one of the basic principles (BP) discussed earlier, which is to keep your feet moving. It is far too easy for a defender to guard a player standing still waiting for a pass. When the player receiving the pass is going across the ice at the blue line there is no ice gained, while they risk missing the pass or getting hit and losing the puck. Even if the player receives the pass, the situation is generally 2 forwards against 2 defenders, and this is not the odd man advantage (BP) we are trying to generate.

The simple break out (Figure C) is for me the best. It gets all offensive players moving together up the ice, hitting the offensive zone together at full speed. If you can get over the blue line carrying the puck and establish your power play positions, then this is preferred. If the defensive wall is strong, not allowing you to carry the puck over the blue line, then get the puck deep to a corner away from the goalie, and get 2 or 3 players on the puck until you regain control and start your power play rotations.

Especially in the younger ages, when penalty kill pressure is applied hard into your zone, both wingers should be back as outlets, and their feet should be moving. This will allow the defenseman to easily start the breakout on either side of the ice. Complicated switching of positions by the forwards, to compensate for forwards staying high, just increases the prospect of the breakout failing. The key point is that the offensive team wants to get the puck out of the zone under control. If a turnover does occur, maximum strength is available to defend and recover the puck quickly.

### Figure C - Power Play Breakout

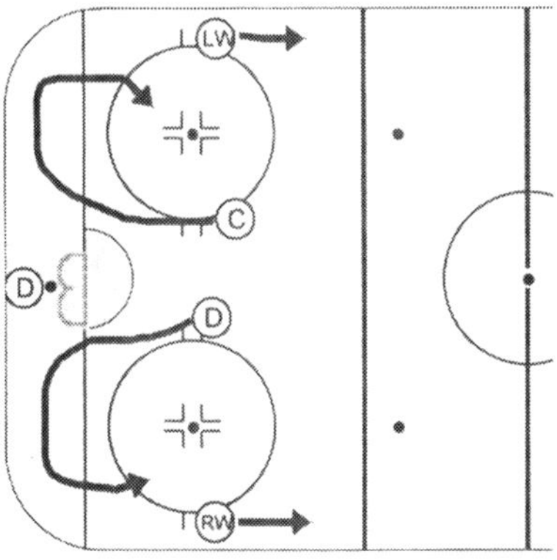

The goal is to get set up with the (D) behind the net and wait for all offensive players to get into position. They can then breakout together with speed.

# 7

# THE PENALTY KILL FORE-CHECK

*Be 100% sure before committing low
in the offensive zone.
Keep control of the center of the ice.
Angle and pressure the puck carrier
to force a pass or a dump in.
Create a defensive wall in the neutral area.
Force the offensive team to dump the puck in
to gain the zone.*

The basics (like all plays there are many variations) come down to an aggressive or passive fore-check.

The passive is the easiest (figure D). It allows the offensive team to leave their zone unchallenged, with the purpose of clogging the neutral area (between the two blue lines). This should simultaneously slow up the offensive rush and hopefully force a turnover. Should the offensive team get to the center line, maximum pressure is available to force the puck to be dumped into the zone therefore giving up control of the puck. The inverted "T" formation puts 3 defenders at their blue line and one player at the tip of the "T". This player's responsibility is to force the puck carrier to the boards, taking away space. This side pressure and defensive wall at the blue line forces the offensive player to have to dump the puck in to gain the zone. This strategy is effective against strong puck handling and passing teams which will take advantage of the penalty killing team being stretched out on an aggressive fore-check (by default generally older players).

The aggressive fore-check (figure E & F) puts pressure on the offensive defensemen in their zone. It forces the defenseman to come out from behind the net, in the direction desired by the lead fore-checker, by blocking one side of the net to escape. The fore-checker should never chase the defenseman behind the net as this will allow the defenseman to move freely out the other side. The defender should try not to commit below the goal line as this creates too much space (stretches the gap between defenders) for the offensive team to move the puck unimpeded. The second forward penalty killer will move like a safety in football, watching the offensive puck carrier's moves, and being ready to move to attack the puck after it has been passed. The low penalty killer, after forcing the initial pass, will continue attacking the puck if the low penalty killer is still closest to the puck after the pass (figure E). If the low penalty killer [F1] forces the initial pass to the left winger (figure F), and is no longer closest to the puck, he should then break off the attack of the puck. The low penalty killer will back check down the middle of the ice to cut off the second pass and take away the center of the ice. The second high forward [F2] will move on an angle to attack the left winger, who has just received the pass, and attempt to stop the play.

The key to the penalty kill fore-check is that there are no center or specific positions for the forwards in the penalty kill. The closest forward to the puck attacks and has that side of the ice, and the other forward takes the center of the ice. Effectively, you are in a penalty kill box position from one end of the ice to the other. The forward in the support role (not attacking the puck) is staggered back from the attacking forward and fills the passing lanes in the middle. If the initial forward is beaten, the second forward, in a position slightly back, must attack the puck carrier on an angle to either side of the ice. The attacker's role is to contain the puck carrier and force the player toward the boards. Attacking the puck carrier, especially at the younger ages, is critical. Every pass has a 50% chance, at most, of success. Pressure causes bad decisions and turnovers. Lastly, you never want an opposing forward going up the ice with speed unchallenged against a young defenseman. The forwards must continue to switch sides, with the closest forward always attacking the puck carrier, taking away the puck carrier's space until the puck moves inside the blue line where the box positions are established.

Some teams employ offensive players out at the far blue line trying to take advantage of the long pass. To defend any stretch pass strategy, teach the defense to face the puck (the other team's end) and station themselves somewhere between the red line and their blue line. They should keep the stretched offensive players behind them as the pass must first go past the defender. They should not chase the forward around or get distracted, and especially should not turn their back on the play. They should swivel their heads and stay in a direct line between the puck carrier and the stretch player. In this way, in the older ages, a hard high pass cannot be made that could be gloved down by the stretch player. In this formation players are still in an extended box formation and have effectively taken two offensive players out of the rush. The short handed team actually has 4 players to the opposition's 3 players closest to the puck. This creates an advantage for the defending team on recovering missed passes and loose pucks. As the play moves up the ice the two defenders move back behind the two stretch offensive players, maintaining a very close gap and trying to force the dump-in.

## Figure D - The Passive Penalty Kill Fore-check

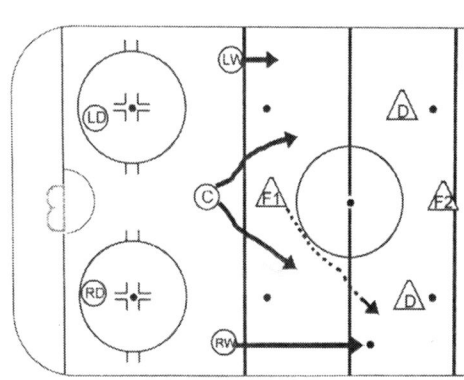

The opposition is allowed to come out of their zone unchallenged, and the lead forward [F1] will steer the puck carrier to either boards. The defense [D], with [F2] in the middle, creates a wall at the blue line forcing the puck to be dumped into the defensive zone.

## Figure E - The Aggressive Penalty Kill Fore-check

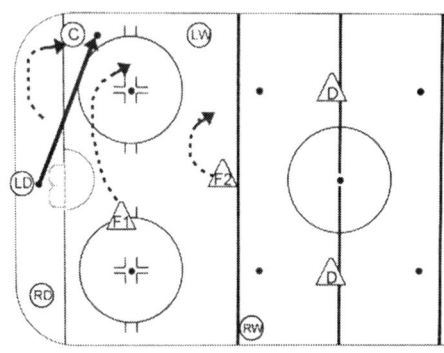

[F1] forces the play to the one side, angling the (LD), applying pressure, and forcing the pass. If [F1] remains closest to the play, then [F1] continues to pursue the puck.

[F2] moves over high to collect turnovers and put immediate pressure on any pass made.

## Figure F - The Aggressive Penalty Kill Fore-check

[F1] forces the play to one side and breaks off pursuit of the puck, as [F2] is now closer to the puck carrier.

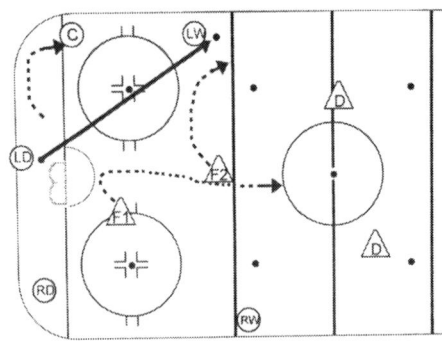

[F1] back checks up the middle of the ice to take away the cross ice pass and to attack the puck if [F1] becomes closer to the puck after [F2]'s attack

# 8

# THE PENALTY KILL BOX IN OUR END

*No one enters the box without pressure.*
*As the puck gets closer to our net*
*the box gets smaller, plugging lanes.*
*Maintain controlled pressure on the puck*
*to force mistakes and turnovers.*
*Active sticks and feet to block passing lanes*
*through the box*
*Don't get tied up with any one player*

Once the puck gets into our zone the defenders in a 4 man system establish a box (Figure G) the two forwards will be high, and the two defensemen will be low. The defenders' prime responsibility is to ensure that the offensive team does not get inside the box, either by carrying the puck or passing to another player close to the net. As the offensive team sets up outside the box, the defensive team works to pressure the puck carrier into a mistake without stretching the box too wide. Stretching the box opens up room for cutting offensive players to gain position in the box, and to improve their chances of scoring. Once the puck carrier is forced to lose control of the puck, or take a bad shot, maximum pressure should be applied by the closest defender to try to recover the puck and ice it. It is critical that all defenders keep their sticks active. Defenders should move their sticks and feet to block all passing lanes while maintaining a body position between the puck and the goalie at all times. Anyone trying to enter the box requires immediate attention. The box, especially the forward positions, must collapse (to [F1] positions) to support the defense when any player enters the box. A shot from outside the box is the only thing your team wants to give up until you have a chance to recover the puck. The box must expand (to [F2] positions) as the puck moves to the point players, and must collapse (to [F1] positions) as the puck gets closer to your net. A puck behind your net may force the defending forwards to drop lower than [F1] if required. The defending forwards will look for offensive players lurking in front of the net just behind the defense. The defensemen must now turn their backs to the front of the net to focus on keeping the puck carrier from coming out in front of the net. As the defensemen cannot see behind themselves, the forwards must be responsible for any intruders into the box. Constant verbal communication is a must amongst all defenders.

As a side note, the issue that defensemen should always stay in front of their net is overrated. It is becoming more common to see constant pressure on the puck carrier as the first priority. A strong rotation from the other defenders is critical to maintaining the defensive box, especially when a defenseman leaves the front of the net unattended to attack the puck carrier. A common offensive power play set up (Figure H) would have a winger with the puck on the boards, center below the goal line on the same side of the ice, and a winger in front of the net. The defending defenseman closest to the puck will jockey back and forth between the two offensive players who are trying to make the defender over-commit. When the puck is moved from the player on the boards to the center below the goal line an opportunity for a bad pass or fumbled pass occurs. The defenseman in front of the net, if now closest to the puck, should move immediately on any poor pass, and should attack the player before the player can recover control of the puck. The defender leaving the offensive player alone in front of the net is not an issue. The top offside forward [F2] will react to the defenseman's move and move lower to the front of the net to cover the offensive forward. The defensive winger near the boards [F1] on the strong side will move to the middle of the ice high. The defender originally in the corner will move toward the front of the net, releasing the forward who has dropped down to go back to his high box position. Effectively, the defensemen have switched positions, while maintaining maximum pressure on the puck (again this should happen during 5 on 5 situations as well). The move by the defenseman should not be made if the offense completes the pass cleanly below the red line. This would allow the offensive player to quickly make a pass out in front of the net for an easy scoring chance before the defensive rotation could take place.

Overall, if the offensive player has control of the puck and their head facing the defender, controlled pressure should be exerted without over committing. Contain the player by staying between the puck and the net. When an offensive player mishandles the puck, or turns his back to the play, then the defender can apply more pressure trying to recover the puck and send it down the ice. Defenders must also realize that when an offensive player is caught alone after recovering a rebound, or due to bad offensive positioning, that this is a good time to apply full pressure and gain control of the puck. If immediate control is not obtained, then the defender should move back to the box and a control position. Too often in minor hockey the offensive team is conducting a change in the offensive zone, and the defenders continue to maintain the box. This allows the offense to keep control outside the box. The players should communicate loudly when an offensive player leaves the zone for any reason. Full pressure should be applied immediately, as you are now 4 on 4.

When defending a 5 on 3 penalty kill, a defensive triangle is established and rotates constantly to try to apply pressure on the puck. Defend the triangle area to ensure no offensive players can get inside the triangle with the puck unless they are under pressure. The biggest mistake seen in minor hockey is one poor forward trying to skate back and forth, from offensive defenseman to offensive defenseman, while both defending defensemen try to take players in front of the net. This allows the offensive defensemen to spread out to evade the one forward. They can then move quickly into the scoring area for a great scoring opportunity. The preferred way to defend on a 5 on 3 is to not get tied up with any one offensive player. The reason for this is simple, as you are already down 2 players, and dedicating one on one makes the odds better for the remaining offensive players. This also helps the offense accomplish the basic principle of creating an odd man advantage. The defenseman-to-defenseman passes (Figure J) should not be defended by the forward defender chasing them across the ice, but by the defending defenseman in front of the net [D2] moving out to challenge the puck carrier. This defenseman moving toward the puck also allows the defender to attempt to block any potential shot. The other defender [D1] slides across to the front of the net. The defending forward [F1] then drops lower to guard the net area and reestablish the triangle. Should the puck be moved back to the other defenseman, then the reverse rotation occurs. Effectively, the closest defender to the puck stays with the puck carrier, and the other two adjust to maintain the most coverage possible in the slot area. Clog the lanes, have active sticks, and block all the shots you can. Remember though, that you can't afford to get tied up with any one player. Always face the puck, taking away as many passing lanes as possible. Anticipate and react quickly to your rotation requirements.

### Figure G - The 4 Player Box

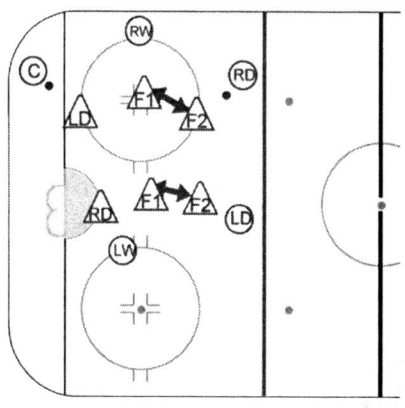

The box when the puck is with (C) down low, the forwards are in [F1] positions collapsed down low.

The box when the puck is with the (D) has the forwards stretched to [F2] positions.

## Figure H - The 4 Player Box Rotations

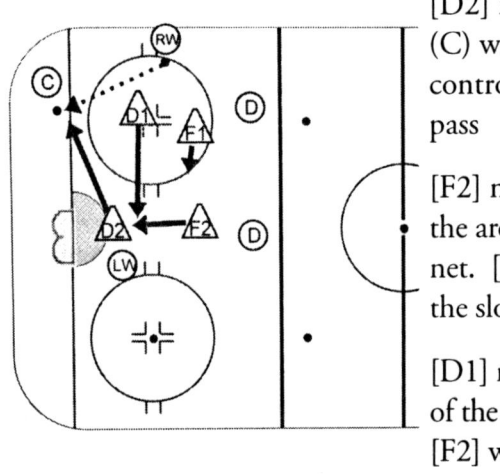

[D2] moves to attack (C) when (C) loses control or receives a bad pass

[F2] moves back to fill the area in front of the net. [F1] collapses to the slot area.

[D1] moves to the front of the net and relieves [F2] with [F1] & [F2] moving to their original box positions.

## Figure J - The 3 Player Triangle Rotations

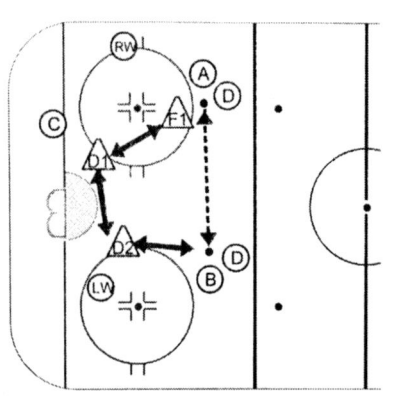

As the puck moves (D) to (D) (between (A) and (B)):

[F1] drops down to [D1].

[D1] moves to the front of the net [D2].

[D2] moves out to puck.

Rotation reverses as puck moves back to (A)

# 9

# 5 Player Fore-check

*You are in defense mode until the puck is freed
from the opposition.
Never get caught deep where one pass
can beat two attackers.
First player in pressures the puck and takes the man.
Second player maintains a support position
and captures the loose puck.
Third player is high to support the defense
on a breakout.
Understand and adjust to the game situation.*

I like to break the game into steps that are easy to remember and therefore easy to teach. The key to an effective fore-check is to get on the puck as quickly as possible with the proper support (Figure K). The first player into the zone has the responsibility to angle the puck carrier and to take the body in contact situations, and in non contact to cut the player off. This effectively frees the puck from the defender. The second player into the zone is in the area below the top of face-off circle. That player is ready to go to the free puck, if the first player succeeds in freeing it, or will hang back to cut off the pass up the boards or through the middle to a cutting centerman should the defender gain control of the puck. The third forward is high in the slot and ready to retreat on the back check if the fore-check fails. In the case of the puck being moved behind the net and out the other side, the third forward will time the fore-check to cut off the play as it comes around behind the net. As the puck moves behind the net, the second forward will move laterally across the ice to take up the second position on the other side of the ice. The first forward does not chase the puck carrier behind the net, but retreats to the high slot ready to back check if required. In all cases, the triangle offense positioning must be maintained to ensure the maximum coverage of the passing and skating lanes. If an offensive defenseman pinches in (usually later in the game when a goal is needed) the high forward will generally cover for the pinching defenseman. It does not have to be the winger on the side of the defenseman, although you see this method being taught by coaches in many amateur games. Generally, the winger on the same side of the pinching defenseman should be deep on the fore-check and is the last person in a position to cover for the defenseman. The key part to the fore-check is to ensure that you have someone high, and that 3 forwards are not trapped deep in the zone. This might lead to a breakout by the opposition which leads to a 3 on 2 (an odd man advantage which goes against the basic principles).

In a situation in which the defenders get to the puck and set up behind their net, it is important not to chase behind the net as this breaks the basic principle (BP) of keeping yourself between the puck and your goal. The low man forces the play to one side of the net or the other, with the remaining forwards taking up positions high at the top of the circle, away from the boards and in line with the face-off dots. Remember, that if the other team sends 3 forwards out of the zone, then the two forwards would set up as far back as necessary to be close to the other forwards but between the forwards and the puck. Only one player chases the puck carrier deep, so that an easier break out, with one pass beating two players, cannot cause an odd man advantage up the ice.

In the final minutes of the game, when holding a lead, the second forward takes up a higher position (known as a 1-2-2). With the other team in control of the puck, the other forwards do not support deep into the opposition's end unless 100% sure of puck recovery. At this time, another goal is not needed, and many games have been lost due to the greed of players trying to pad their stats and getting caught down low in the offensive end. A player taking a bad chance (even if a goal is scored) should not be congratulated without a strong reprimand for selfish play. Emphasize that the team must come first, and the responsibility of playing in the last few minutes of any game goes to the players who recognize and play to the team values. A player taking a shot at an open net from their side of the red line risks an icing call and a resulting face-off in their own zone. The players must be taught to work to cross the red line before any shot attempt. If the red line cannot be crossed, then the puck should be angled off the boards to take off some speed on hard clearing shots, or the puck should be dumped with enough

## Figure K - Five Player Fore-check

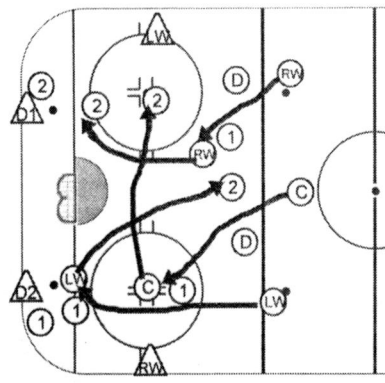

Players attack puck in corner (1).
First player (LW) into zone goes to the puck.
Second player (C) comes in to support around dot.
Third Player (RW) stays high on weak side.

As play is shifted to other side (2),
(RW) is now closest to the puck and moves to cut off puck carrier.
(C) moves across ice to support at dot.
(LW) breaks off and moves back to high position.

# 10

# 5 Player Defensive Positioning in Our End
# (the centerman's role)

*Similar to the penalty kill box with
an attacking player closest to the puck
Keep your eyes on the puck and the player
being covered at all times.
Collapse the box to support attacks into the box.
Keep the puck outside the box.
Wingers are responsible for the offensive defensemen.*

Most coaches and spectators know that when you are killing a penalty with 4 players you are positioned in a box, and the goal is to keep the opposition outside of the box. Why is it then that you never hear, during 5 on 5 situations, someone yelling from the bench or stands to "Box it up!"? The 5 man defensive strategy in your own zone is simply a 4 man box with the player closest to the puck aggressively attacking the puck carrier (Figure L). This is not an odd man advantage situation. If the other team has 2 on the puck, then so should you. If they have 3 then put 3. Remember the basic principles. Stay between the puck and your goalie. Never fight for a puck on the boards unless you have body control of the offensive player. Too many times you see the defensive player take a position against the boards to try to dislodge the puck from the skates of a player who is pinning the puck to the boards. The puck is freed, but the offensive player pivots off the boards and wins the race to the puck. This generally leads to a good scoring chance. This can also happen to the second defensive player into the battle on the boards. A freed puck can easily end up on the stick of the offensive player left open because the second defensive player entered the pile of players to poke at the puck. Contain all players by keeping them in front of you, and take the face-off if necessary.

As the offensive team moves the puck inside your zone from the corner (figure L) - to the point (figure M) - the defensive player [RW] closest to the puck will aggressively attack the puck carrier. Communication (BP) is critical, so that only one player is attacking the puck carrier at any time. The other players are rotating within the defensive zone box, picking up one of the 4 corners of the box. The box is always maintained, and one player is always attacking the puck. The box will continue to stretch and float based on the positioning of the offensive players, and all defenders should be within stick reach of the player they are covering in their area of the box. As shown in figure M, the box is stretched, as the center [C] is closer to the (LW) on the boards, and the [D] has dropped lower with body position between the net and the offensive center. As in the penalty kill box, the offensive players should be kept outside the box.

Once the puck is recovered, and only then, do the forwards and defense partners spread out to the boards to start the break out. Should the breakout fail, and the puck is lost, the players should react as quickly as possible to reestablish their box positions and pick up their assignments. A key to defending your end is the high forward pair. They are responsible for covering the offensive defenseman, and therefore should not be in the corners or behind the net. As the puck moves lower in the zone the box collapses lower, and it opens up as the puck moves higher. Positioning of the defending players is critical, as you are not covering the player man for man. The defender must always be in a position to see the puck and the player they are covering (the defender's back is to the middle of the box). This will ensure that the player being covered does not cut to an open spot behind your back. With this positioning, passes will be made by the offensive players outside the box, but as long as the box is not penetrated the defense is working effectively. If the player's reaction did not allow them to cut off the pass, then they should attack the puck carrier aggressively, keeping their body between the puck and the net. They have support behind them in the form of the box.

Too many times you see the defending forwards too high in the coverage of the offensive defenseman. This is a mistake, as an offensive forward may beat a defender and will have a clear lane to the scoring area before the defensive wingers can drop down in support. The roles of the top defending wingers are to challenge the offensive defensemen, block shots from the point, and to force the play outside. The primary role is to support the box, collapsing lower as the puck moves lower towards the goal line and not allowing entry into the box. This means that if one of the defenders gets beaten, the other defenders must collapse the box to take away the entry lanes and reestablish the wall until the defender that was beaten can rejoin the box. An offensive player inside the box area, who is not covered by a defenseman, must receive attention from the defending forwards. A shot from outside the box or from the point is preferred to a shot coming from right in front of your net. The defenders must read the situation and rotate their defensive positioning to take away the most probable passing lanes. Take a position close to any offensive player inside the box, as they are most likely the highest risk to score if the puck gets to them.

*Hockey For Parents*

## Figure L - Five Player Box –Puck in the Corner

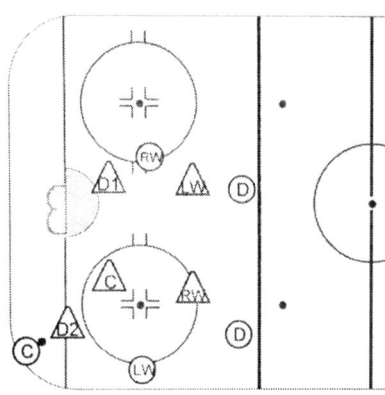

[D2] attacks the puck carrier (C) under control.

[C] is in a support position to recover the puck if [D2] is successful in dislodging it or to cover for [D2] if beaten.

[LW] and [RW] are lower, collapsing the box as the puck is below the goal line.

## Figure M - Five Player Box – Puck at the Point

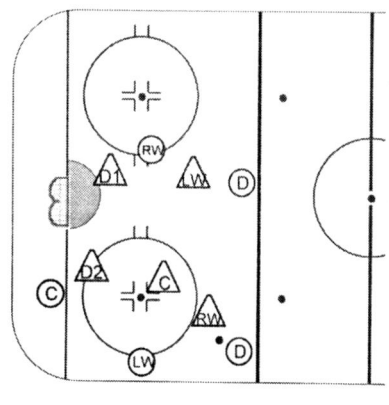

[RW] attacks the puck carrier, with [C] acting as support, staying at the height of the opposing (LW) on the boards as this is the next logical pass.

[LW] moves out toward (D), but not far enough to allow (D) to cut past the [LW] into the box, or stretching the box too much.

# 11

## FACE-OFFS IN THE DEFENSIVE END

*One defenseman on the boards*
*Winger moves inside on a path to the offensive defenseman on the boards.*
*Other winger attacks other offensive defenseman.*
*Centerman takes Centerman after draw.*
*Defenseman in front of net takes opposing winger.*

There are two basic but separate face-off alignments. One would be used for experienced teams, and one for younger teams. In both cases the center does not prepare to take the face-off until all the defenders are in their correct positions based on the offensive team's alignment.

Let's focus on the experienced team's alignment in the circle to the right of their goal. All players have a defined role. They need to act quickly at the drop of the puck to get into their defensive positions discussed in the 5 man defensive end coverage. The focus of all defenders is to anticipate the drop of the puck by watching the official's hand movement. They should commence movement as soon as the official releases the puck, not when it hits the ice.

The center is responsible for winning the face-off backward towards the boards and into corner. No matter what happens on the draw, win or lose, the opposing center is the defending center's responsibility until the defenders gain control or neutralize the immediate offensive threat of a lost draw. The defenders, at the drop of the puck, are moving to their assignments in the 5 man box formation. For clarification on a common mistake, the center should not go to the point on lost draws, but remain with the offensive center. This may require the center to move away from the puck, if necessary, to maintain contact with the opposing center. This is a common defensive error on a lost draw usually resulting in the offensive center being left uncovered and deflecting a shot, or scoring on a rebound.

The left winger is established in front of the net at the hash marks and outside of the right defenseman. The sole purpose is for the left winger to move out to the offensive right point player and establish the left side of the box (figure N). If the draw is won, then the left winger breaks off to the left boards (figure P), around the hash marks of the left circle, and prepares for the break out. At a senior level on won draws, the [LW] may break out of the zone for a long stretch pass from their defenseman if the offensive defenseman in the middle of the ice is committed too low on the face-off.

The right winger moves to the left side of the circle and to the right of the right defenseman, generally a step below the hash marks. The target route is from this inside position on the left side of the circle, to move directly towards the offensive left defenseman. The right winger has three responsibilities on lost draws (figure N) while on this route. These happen in sequence. The first responsibility is to take the puck, if the draw has come toward the player, progress with it out of the zone or send the puck to safety in the corner. This creates the same result as if the draw had been won on the face-off. The second responsibility, on a short draw when the puck goes directly behind the offensive centerman is to go to the offensive left winger if this player is coming around behind or started behind the centerman on the draw. Make the hit or relieve the left winger of the puck. The third responsibility is on a clean long draw back to the offensive left defenseman is while advancing to the point to block any shot taken. Players should be taught to apply direct and immediate pressure on the defenseman, and to finish their checks. After a draw, until the defensive team gains control, the right winger moves on route and stops at the top right side of the defensive box (if the puck does not go to the left defenseman). On a won draw the right winger (Figure P) starts on their route and then diverts to the right boards as a breakout option for the defenseman. If the puck is wrapped around behind the net to the left winger, then the right winger can continue skating up ice and can clear the zone looking for a breakaway stretch pass.

The left defenseman (assuming the player shoots left) takes the position at the right of the circle on the hash marks. Switching is not recommended if both defensemen shoot the same way as no advantage is gained, and the defense will start in their off positions. This defenseman must be high on the hash marks to pressure the offensive left winger, not in the corner. This will force the offensive centerman to win the face-off backwards to maintain control and not to simply draw the puck sideways to their winger. The first movement of the left defenseman is toward the face-off dot on the low side of their center. On a won draw to the corner, this defenseman peels to retrieve the puck. This positioning allows the defenseman to be the first to the puck and to commence the breakout. On lost draws that go directly to the boards (figure N) the right defenseman should battle the winger to win control of the puck, while all other players move to their box positions. On a lost draw that goes toward the blue line or short behind the offensive centerman, the defenseman comes below the center and establishes the lower box position. This point is critical because even if the offensive winger on the boards has control and is proceeding behind their centerman for a shot, the defenseman does not pursue and still goes below the center, back to the low post position. The job of the right winger coming through ([RW] point 2 of his route) is to take the puck carrier before the player clears their centerman and can release a shot. On won draws, (figure P) the defensemen are switched to ensure that the defenseman on the boards is on their forehand so that they can clear the puck around the boards behind the net to the left winger. This will start the break out or allow the winger to tip the wrap around pass and clear the zone. The left defenseman, given time, can carry the puck behind the net and stop, or carry on behind the net to start the breakout. The other option is to reverse the play and go up the right boards which should now have the right winger awaiting a pass after breaking off their initial route.

The right defenseman takes the position in front of the net (figure N) switching with his defense partner with sole responsibility of covering the offensive right winger. The right defenseman moves along the hash marks to remain opposite the right winger wherever that player lines up. If the offensive right winger goes wide away from the face-off dot, and the right offensive defenseman moves in closer, then the defending right defenseman and left winger must communicate and switch starting positions. This will ensure that the defending left winger is now closer to the face-off dot, and defenders are now closer to their assigned players. On a won draw, (figure P), the right defenseman can move to accept a breakout pass behind the net or in the opposite corner and generally will move to support the left side on the breakout.

For younger teams I recommend a different alignment for the following reasons which effectively focus on a strong wall between the face-off dot and the goalie.

At the younger ages the defensemen generally do not have strong enough shots to be a threat to score directly off the draw. The offensive centerman is generally a strong player who, on the face-off, is more likely to go forward than to draw the puck backward. The defensive wingers and defensemen are learning their positions, and therefore it is best not to put them in switched or off-wing situations to avoid unnecessary confusion.

The structure for the younger teams is a simple face-off set up at the left dot (figure Q). The left winger is on the left boards beside the offensive right winger. The center should take the opposing center, and the defensive right winger goes to the left point. The left defenseman lines up behind and to the right of center at 4 o'clock. The left defenseman has the sole responsibility of taking any puck coming back from the draw or pushed forward by the opposing center. The player's first movement should be forward into the circle with the single purpose of getting to the puck, or taking the offensive center coming toward the net. The left defenseman acts as a rover and has the sole responsibility of picking up all loose pucks off the draw. Each defender on the line is responsible for taking the person beside them. This allows the defenseman as much time as possible to collect the puck. By being quick off the draw, players can position their bodies in front of the offensive players without interfering. This positioning will force the offensive player to skate around them, lengthening the time to get to the puck. The right defenseman's role is unchanged and entails taking the offensive left winger in front of the net.

In a different situation, the offensive team might move their right winger in front of the net or behind the center. In this case, the defensive left winger must move to the right side of the face-off circle in front of the net with the sole purpose of lining up to take that offensive right winger once the puck drops. The left winger is moved to the front of the net to ensure that the left winger stays between the goalie and the player they are to defend (BP). The winger on the boards is taught to evaluate the offense positioning prior to the face-off. If lining up on the boards would not have them beside an opponent, then they will line up in front of the net. Players must communicate with their teammates so that everyone agrees on their assignments before the puck drops. It is critical that centermen are taught that they should not line up to take the face-off until all teammates are in their correct defensive positions.

Refer to the basics when discussing any face-off alignment with your child. Any defensive alignment which does not have a player positioned in a direct line between the puck, or player being covered and the goalie (BP) is a weak alignment. A commonly seen weak alignment has a left defenseman placed in the left corner to receive the draw. This alignment puts the defenseman in a starting position that is not between the puck, or the player they are assigned to defend, and the goal. As this goes against the basic principles I would not recommend this alignment.

*Hockey For Parents*

## Figure N - Face-off lost draw our end

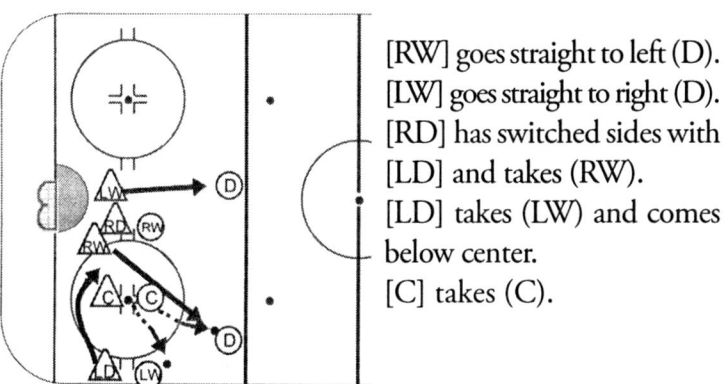

[RW] goes straight to left (D).
[LW] goes straight to right (D).
[RD] has switched sides with [LD] and takes (RW).
[LD] takes (LW) and comes below center.
[C] takes (C).

## Figure P-Face-off won draw our end

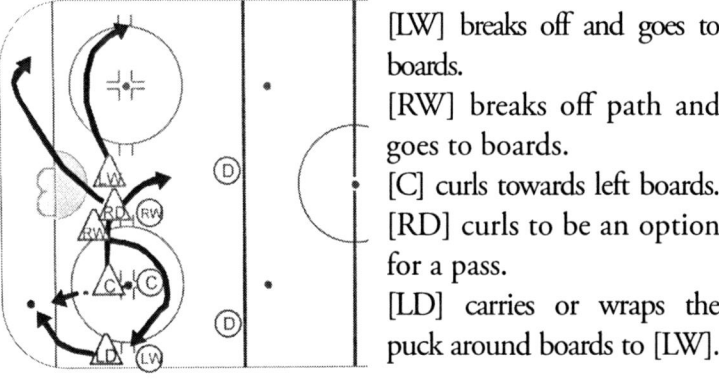

[LW] breaks off and goes to boards.
[RW] breaks off path and goes to boards.
[C] curls towards left boards.
[RD] curls to be an option for a pass.
[LD] carries or wraps the puck around boards to [LW].

## Figure Q-Face-off for younger teams

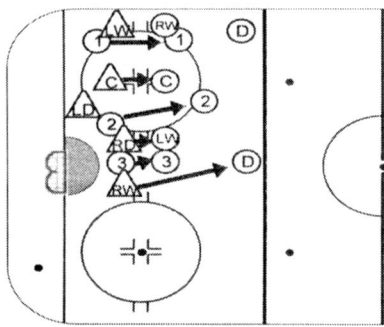

Defensive [LW] will line up in position (1, 2, 3) to match wherever offensive (RW) lines up (1, 2, 3).

[LD] low is responsible for all loose pucks on draw and for stopping opposing center.

# 12

## Face-offs in the Offensive End

*Have a plan going in for where the draw is to go.*
*Maintain maximum pressure in alignment*
*in case of a lost draw.*
*Anticipate the drop of the puck.*
*Get the shot past the oncoming defenders*
*even if you miss the net.*

Understanding all the points made in the defensive face-off structure, it is now up to the offensive team to alter their alignments to try to confuse the defenders. Hopefully with this confusion, the defenders will miss their assignments, and a scoring chance can be generated. I believe that if the defenders follow the routes and responsibilities stated earlier, only a quick shot or initial control should be achieved. The offensive goal is to take advantage of the defenders' mistakes.

As there are so many offensive face-off alignments, I will not go into all the different variations, but I would like to focus on a few glaring errors that take away the advantage of having a face-off in the opposing zone. Remember, that before the center enters the circle, it is their responsibility to ensure that all the offensive players are aligned the way the center wants. The center will attempt to draw the puck to a set area of the ice that is best for this offensive alignment. Let's use the right offensive circle as our example to discuss some potential errors made on offensive face-offs.

Let's agree that the goal of any face-off is to win the draw and gain control of the puck. It is therefore imperative that in a manner similar to football, the quarterback (your defenseman) must have as much time as possible to make the right decision. To this end, the aim on the face-off is to make the defending player, who is standing beside you, take the toughest route possible to get to the puck. With the new interference rules, the ability to impede a player is greatly reduced, but all players are entitled to their space on the ice. A center, who wins the draw and turns to face the puck in the path of the defender, or who skates causing a defender to take a longer route to the puck, is legal. The key, especially for the wingers, is to get in the lanes of the wingers pushing out to the point making them go around you.

The offensive defenseman positioning is critical. The basic rule is that the defenseman on the boards is the target for the draw and should be slightly closer to the center. Too often I see the left defenseman in tight to the circle, waiting to get the puck on the draw for a shot. This is extremely dangerous and not recommended, as a lost draw, with the defensive right winger breaking out to the point, will leave the winger open ice behind the defenseman. The winger can now receive a direct pass, a bounce pass off the boards, or a dump pass, any of which put the winger on a clear breakaway. The right offensive defenseman on the boards is not in a position to stop a breaking forward, as the basic principle of being between your goal and the puck has been lost. This low positioning of the left defenseman also makes it very difficult, on a lost draw, for the defenseman to react to the defenders wrapping the puck around to the winger on the far boards and stopping the breakout. On a face-off on this side of the ice, the left offensive defenseman has to be thinking defensively and to be the first player back on a lost draw. If the draw is won, the movement to offense will happen instinctively and quickly.

Some teams employ a strategy of taking the right offensive winger off the boards and either moving this player in front of the net or into a shooting position on the top of the circle. In this circumstance the offensive team has made a key strategic error. They have allowed the defending center to move the puck to the unprotected area toward the boards. The defending defenseman can then easily commence the breakout, or clear the puck from the zone. This alignment has actually created space for the defense (BP) which is not to the offenses' advantage. If the winger is the player with the stronger shot, then the right offensive defender should move down to within a stick length or two of the defending player on the boards, and this defenseman must be given permission to commit lower to play the puck if the draw is lost in that direction. On the loss of the draw, with this positioning, the right offensive winger must react to the lost draw and move back quickly to fill the right offensive defenseman's position at the point.

Another common mistake occurs on a won draw back to the defense. The defense will be taking a shot with defenders charging at them, and if the defenders are doing it right they will be on a line between their goal and the puck. The shooting defenseman must therefore ensure that their shot gets past the defender, even if it means missing the net. The other defenseman, who is not taking the shot, must always be prepared for the shot to be blocked and should be moving back outside the blue line to recover the puck or to defend against an attack should the defenders recover the blocked shot.

# 13

## HOW TO CORRECTLY EXECUTE A 2 ON 1

*The player with the puck drives wide,*
*then directly to the net.*
*If the defenseman comes, then pass.*
*If not, then drive to the net and score.*
*The player without the puck must create a lane*
*to receive the pass.*
*Both players drive for the rebound- don't turn off.*
*Only pass if it improves the chance to score.*

The 2 on 1 is one of the most exciting plays in hockey. It is also the most over-thought and most often wasted advantage. The offensive players continue to complicate this basic play by forcing a pass, as opposed to simply reading and reacting to the defending player. The basic and simple rules for a 2 on 1 are as follows. The player with the puck enters the zone wide and drives to the net reading the defenseman's intentions. If the defenseman comes to the puck, the player passes, and if not, the player drives unimpeded to the net similar to a break away. The player without the puck must establish a speed and pacing to ensure that, at any time, there is a clear lane to receive the pass. This is done by slowing up or speeding past the defender on the way to the goal area. A lane for the pass must be maintained to deter the defenseman from attacking the puck carrier. Frequently, as soon as a player with the puck crosses the blue line on a 2 on 1, the crowd starts yelling at the poor puck carrier to pass. They continue to yell, even when there is little or no chance of completing the pass as the lone defender (who is anticipating the pass) has moved beside the player without the puck. Why should any player pass the puck if the player is feeling no defensive pressure and therefore is effectively on a clear cut breakaway? They should not. Until that defenseman commits to stopping the puck carrier, the puck carrier should continue to drive to the net. Parents, please stop yelling for the puck carrier to pass. Too many opportunities are missed when a puck carrier without pressure tries to pass the puck to a covered teammate instead of driving to the net and taking a shot. If the shot does not lead to a goal, then a rebound will be available for the other forward going to the net. On driving to the net, if the defenseman reacts late to the puck carrier, in today's rules a holding or hooking penalty to the defender is a common positive result. If the defenseman does commit late to the puck carrier, then an easy cross ice pass for an open net goal is also available, as the goalie must commit to the puck carrier.

Therefore parents please revise the coaching from the stands. Players should not pass until the time is right. The player should drive the net and read the defenseman. Passing is the second option, if the defenseman takes away the first option of driving the net. If the puck carrier doesn't drive the net for a scoring opportunity and goes wide, then the defender can focus on the open player, effectively taking away the passing option.  This will most likely stop all chances to score on this rush.  So the new yell from the stands should be "**Drive the Net!**"

# 14

## How To Correctly Execute a 3 on 2

*First player over the blue line takes the puck wide and drives to the net.*
*Second player drives the net for the pass.*
*Third player stays high for the pass.*
*Communicate by yelling I am 1, I am 2, or I am 3.*
*Create space and passing lanes.*

Similarly to the 2 on 1, the focus is to get the puck to the net for the best possible scoring opportunity. The basic rules for a 3 on 2 are simple and if followed consistently create the best scoring opportunities. The position being played is irrelevant to executing a successful 3 on 2. It is simply 3 offensive players working to spread out the 2 defenders. I see many coaches telling forwards that the winger goes wide, the center stays high, and the other winger drives the net. The problem with giving instructions that use specific positions and give defined responsibilities for a 3 on 2 is that all players are not in identical positions as they cross the blue line. Basic rules and teachings have to be flexible to allow for the flow of play, and to take into account the fact that each player will hit the blue line at a different time on individual rushes. Odd man opportunities are what we work to create throughout the game, so to mess up a 3 on 2 may make the difference between team success and failure. The basics of executing the 3 on 2 correctly would have the first player (carrying the puck from any position) going over the opponent's blue line wide of a defender, and then driving on a path toward the corner of the net. If the first player to the blue line is the center, then the aim is still to take the puck to the outside. The winger on that side will switch and move to the middle of the ice surface. The second player (no matter what their position) over the blue line drives the net forcing the opposing defenseman to go with them. The third player over the line should stay high in the slot thus creating the maximum distance from the second forward. This gives the puck carrier two potential pass receivers. The defenders are now split as to which players to cover, and the maximum options have been created to generate a great scoring opportunity. If no one goes to the puck carrier, then that player should "PASS" right (sorry I couldn't resist) or maybe correctly should **"Drive the Net"** just like in the 2 on 1 discussion. If the pressure comes, then find the open player, as the other defender can not cover 2 people at once if the offensive players are properly spaced. Someone must be open. It is critical that the two players without the puck, after spreading out, position themselves to create lanes to receive the pass. Too many times you see that the player trying to receive the pass is not positioned with a clear lane to receive the pass, and the pass is either picked off or made off target. When a shot is taken, all players should drive the net and look for the rebound, reacting to the loose puck. Generally, the third player into the zone will assume the defensive third player high position in case the puck is turned over.

# 15

## Playing Defense. The Toughest Job in Hockey.

*Body position is between the puck and your net.*
*Contain the attacker.*
*Don't commit in the opposite direction.*
*Communicate and use your partner.*
*Control the "gap" between the defense*
*and your forwards.*
*Force the play to the boards.*

Defense is one of the most important and most difficult positions to play in hockey, and yet little instruction and time is dedicated to the defense. Everyone wants to see goals scored, and therefore focus goes naturally to the forwards. Coaches do break-outs during which they dump the puck in for the defense to pick up and make the initial pass, but then watch the forwards bomb up the ice having fun trying to score on 1 or 2 defenders. Too few coaches incorporate the defense as offensive players in the 2 on 1 or 3 on 2 drills. If the defense is taught the proper reactions required on an odd man rush, they will perform better and more team scoring chances will occur. Parents should approach coaches to ensure that the defense will receive equal training and focus prior to the start of the year. On average, 10 to 15 minutes of each practice should be dedicated to the defense. Yes, defending the break out, and a 2 on 1 are very necessary skills and time is well spent on these points, but the defense should be separated from the forwards regularly to focus on defense-specific drills.

**How does a player start a break out while dealing with 3 angry forwards approaching, and knowing that painful physical contact is likely to follow?** How do you angle yourself to take the hit, protect the puck, and move the puck quickly and accurately? Communication is the key. By communicating, "Man On", "Wrap it around the boards", "I am open" (for a D to D pass), the defender on the puck is getting useful information from their partner and the goalie. The goalie plays a large part in controlling the play on the dump-in, from playing the puck, to putting the puck in a position behind the net to give the defenseman the safety of the net, but mostly by being the eyes for the defensemen who have their backs to the attacking players. This communication goes along way to improving the safety and success of controlling the puck and starting the break out. Goalies that push the puck into the corner, or do not come out to play the puck, are leaving the defensemen to take unnecessary hits, and this is not acceptable even at a very young age. Even if it results in the goalie being caught out of position on occasion, the goalie has to be encouraged to play the puck. Practice time for goalies, to learn how to control the puck, pass the puck, and communicate with the defense, will assist the goalie in earning the respect of the defensemen. That respect will go a long way with the defensemen who are asked every game to protect that same goalie.

**How to pass D to D and when to do it?** Passing between defensemen to create space from the oncoming forwards will allow the defense the time necessary to make the proper breakout pass. This will enable them to relieve pressure away from a focused attack to one side of the ice surface. But where does the other D go to be an outlet to best assist their partner who is collecting the puck? When does the player go to the corner? When does the player stay in front of the net? When does he cross over, switching sides of the ice, or utilize a drop or bounce pass to change directional flow of the game? The key, again, is communication by both defensemen, especially the player without the puck. This player should be in a position to receive the pass and should only call for the puck if the passing lane is clear. If the lane is not clear the message should be, "NO, NO, NO!" The defenseman with the puck should then realize a play must be made without a D to D pass. The other key to a D to D pass is that the player without the puck should be slightly behind the puck carrier (closer to their end). This opens up the maximum room for the pass to be made, and also puts the defender in a position to support should their partner lose the puck or make a poor pass. Once the pass is made, the passer will work to get lower again (closer to their end) than their partner for the return pass. When a D to D pass is received, players' feet should already be moving to start up ice or to move the puck to a teammate if open. If no one is open, and there is not open ice, the puck carrier should not panic. The player should look to return the puck to their partner, or to control the puck until options become available.

**When do you pinch in on the offensive boards, and when do you pull out?** What is the responsibility of the other defenseman when this is occurring, and what role does the high forward have? The game situation is also a big factor in determining the action of the defenseman, as more aggression is good when down a goal, but aggression and increasing risk may be foolish when leading. A pinch, or aggressive move into the offensive zone to get the puck, or to body check an opponent, should only be attempted if it has a 90% chance of success and has a high back checking forward for support. Once the offense has the puck under control and is starting to carry the puck, or has teammates moving out of the zone available for a pass, then the defense should leave their positions inside the blue line and start to retreat, maintaining tight "Gap" control with the lead attacking forwards.

**When do you switch positions with your defensive partner?** "Switching" is a term used when the defensemen trade sides of the ice. This is necessitated when one of the defensemen is closer to the puck and can get to the puck more quickly than the other defenseman. It will occur when one defenseman is drawn from the front of the net to attack the puck carrier down low, and the other defenseman rotates back to the front of the net. It is also done intentionally on face-offs, to get the player with the correct handed shot in the best position to succeed after the draw. In all cases it is critical that the defensemen communicate their intentions by yelling, "Switch!" to ensure that both sides of the ice remain covered.

**How do you take a player out in front of your net?**
Taking the offensive player in front of your net is all about body position and control of the opponent's stick. This skill requires practice drills utilizing body position, ensuring the defender always faces the puck (BP) with two hands on the stick. These drills also teach the proper spacing to avoid getting too close to opponents, thus allowing the player to spin into an advantageous position. The key to accomplishing this is to ensure that the defenseman takes a defensive position between the net and the player being covered. You hear people talking about staying between the player and the net at all times. You also hear that to avoid interference penalties due to the new rules, players have to take a position in front of offensive player negating the entry pass. Both statements are correct depending on the situation. The simple way to explain it to your child is to draw a line from the middle of the net straight out between the hash marks. Every offensive player on the puck side of the line should be covered, with the defender between the player and the net (the offensive player in front of you). The defenders should hold their ground, stick on stick, when a shot or pass is

coming. They should move the offensive player away from the net, reducing their angle to shoot or deflect a shot. On the side of the line away from the puck, the defender should be in front of the offensive player. This means that the defending player is still between the offensive player and the net even if the defender is in front of the offensive player. The defending player then backs into the offensive player, moving the player further away from the net. This creates room in front of the net to clear rebounds if necessary. In both cases the defender attempts to move the offensive player further away from the goal and away from the front of the net. This will also give the goalie the best opportunity of seeing the puck without being screened. The key to defending in front of the net is stick on stick, two hands on the stick, and maintaining an arm's length distance from the offensive player. This allows the player to back away on a spin move and not lose positional advantage. Always have knees bent ready to react. Quick rebounds and deflections are all generated from offensive players getting their stick on the puck quickly. That is why defenders in front of the net, and in any battle for the puck, must battle with two hands on the stick. Without two hands on the stick in front of the net, the ability to use strength and speed to clear rebounds is greatly reduced. Remember that controlling the body of the offensive player is very important, but not controlling the stick is the biggest mistake made by most defensemen.

**How do you attack an offensive player in your zone?** Attacking an offensive player in your zone involves quickly assessing the situation. Although each situation requires a different reaction (hockey is all read-and-react, remember), the defender must be taught to look for two basic situations. In a situation in which the offensive player has control of the puck and head up, then a **controlled attack (containment)** is required. Using proper angling of the offensive player, the defender approaches and closes the gap between the two until they are a stick length apart. At this time the defender's job is to try to contain the player as close to the boards as possible, creating enough pressure to cause the player to move the puck or to temporarily lose control. This must be accomplished without getting beaten to the net. If the pressure applied causes puck control to be lost, or the offensive player drops their head to look for the puck, then a more **aggressive attack** should be taken. Approaching at an angle, the player should close the gap immediately, stick on stick, to dislodge the puck, and then should use body contact to remove the player from the puck so it can be recovered by the defender or a teammate. If the defender is not sure that an attack will be successful, the defender should always focus on containment. Jumping at a forward and getting beaten to the net is not a result that will make the coach happy.

**Who is responsible to stop a shot on net?** The Goalie must focus on the puck and be responsible for the initial shot. The defender covering the puck carrier must also do everything possible to block the shot, using correct body position as discussed earlier. A shot on net from the point, that misses the initial block attempt causes a lot of trouble for the defenders. Offensive players should be coming from everywhere to go to the net for a deflection or a rebound. In this situation, the defenders need to be taught that the shot is the responsibility of the goalie. All defenders must rotate their heads and pick up any offensive players coming into the scoring area (the box). This requires defenders taking up the proper defensive position between the net and the offensive player, with stick on stick. Too many times the puck goes to the point, and all attention goes to the puck. This allows players to slip in behind the defenders for an easy deflection or rebound goal. The basic premise to explain this to the defenders is that the puck will not score on its own, so don't worry about it. Concentrate on the possible shooters. A simple game to illustrate this point can be played in your living room or garage. Positioning yourself between your child and the puck, ask your child to get to the puck while you maintain your position between the two. Continue to ask, "Has the puck moved yet?" over and over. This will emphasize that the puck does not score on its own. The key to this exercise is, if you control the offensive player with body position and stick on stick, you will be successful. The goalie, with time, will easily find a rebound and cover it for a face-off.

**How do you block shots correctly?** Blocking shots is cheered loudly in the stands because most people appreciate the courage it takes to stand willingly in front of a slap shot, even with proper equipment. So why do we ask kids to make this brave play and never use practice time to teach the proper techniques? As most kids are now wearing full face masks there are two key points to be taught. First, the majority of equipment protection is on the front of a player. So the player should always face the shot, preferably in the standing position. They should always get as close to where the shot is initiated as possible. This will help increase the probability that the puck will hit the shin pads and not the upper torso or head. In the case of a long shot that could hit the upper torso or head, the chin must be kept down on the chest protecting the throat area. This is also critical when dropping to the ice in front of a shot. The exposed throat area is the most vulnerable area on the player, especially if a puck is deflected upwards. A player should be careful not to reach out, with their stick in front of their body, in an attempt to block a shot. The player may deflect the puck up into the upper body, neck or head. As players get older, more pressure is placed by the coaches to blocking shots at all costs. This makes it critical that practice time be dedicated to proper techniques. These should involve timing of when to hit the ice as the shot is being struck, and of ensuring that only the lower body is presented to the path of the puck. Bravery should not be confused with stupidity. It is very unwise to leave your feet to block a shot far away from the shooter, as this reduces your ability to control where the puck will strike you. If in doubt, stand up, chin down, and with both feet on the ice. Attempting to block a shot with one foot on the ice exposes the unprotected part of the top of the elevated skate. It also looks like the player is afraid of getting hit, so it is not recommended.

**What does staggering mean?** If players are in the offensive zone, the defenseman on the side of the puck near the boards is inside the blue line. The other defenseman must be ready to move outside the offensive zone near the center dot in a support position if the other team gains control on their partner's side of the ice. This is referred to as staggering (supporting your partner 10 to 15 feet behind and on an angle in the middle of the ice). It is critical in lower age groups, as players are more easily beaten during a one on one situation. This staggered position allows the other defenseman to be in a position to recover a loose puck, or to attack the offensive player who has moved past their partner. As the players get older the stagger distance reduces, as pinching or staying inside the blue line is greatly reduced to avoid odd man rushes. The older defensemen will create a straighter wall of defense. This will not allow an offensive player the chance to beat one defender at a time if they are too far apart in a stagger. The older defensemen are also more experienced, physically stronger, and more comfortable in containing an offensive player in a one on one situation. They do not need the support that a younger defenseman may require. The focus of the older defenseman, who is not on the puck carrier, must be on the open opposition players on the other side of the rink, as the skill of passing is high, and the goalie is focused on the puck. Any completed pass will have the goalie out of position and forced to move quickly which increases the offense's chance to score.

**How do you play the one-on-one?** Playing the one-on-one is a recurring situation for all defensemen. This play separates the good defensemen from the soon to be forwards. Again, you hear the basic instructions coming from the stands or from the bench to "watch the chest," or "play the body". Let's first review the basics and see what else is required to be successful. **First**, the most important skill is to match the speed of the oncoming forward. Going too fast will have the defender backing up into their own goal area, allowing the player to shoot from a good scoring area by using the defender as a screen. Backing up too slowly will allow the offensive player to use their speed around the outside to beat the defender. As a side note, once a defender determines that their backward speed is too slow to match the oncoming offensive player, the defender must turn immediately forward and utilize angling techniques. Players must put pride aside and turn as soon as they realize that their speed is not sufficient. This will help avoid those ugly hooking and holding penalties that would otherwise be sure to come. **Second**, body position is critical when skating backward. The offensive player should be positioned on the outside shoulder of the defender, with the intention of forcing the attacking player to the outside toward the boards. Once an angle can be achieved (never slow and then move forward to attempt a hit), turn, close the gap, and then make the hit. Be patient and use the corner of the boards in your end, if necessary, to force the offensive player back to you. **Third**, once the defender's speed is right and the body is in good position, the defender must allow the offensive player to gradually come to them, preferably around the blue line. Forcing the offensive player to shift along the blue line could potentially cause a teammate to go offside. Playing to meet the offensive player as far away from the net as possible reduces the chance of screening the goalie should the offensive player try to shoot. **Fourth**, the defenseman should have the stick held in one hand out in front the defender. This should be aggressively used to knock the puck off the offensive player's stick, or to cause the offensive player to drop their head to fend off the stick or find a dislodged puck. The defender's head should be focused on the offensive player's body at all times, ensuring that good body position is being maintained. Peripheral vision is then used to put the stick in a position to attempt to dislodge the puck from the offensive player's stick. There is a key to your stick position that is often missed. A stick should not be waved wildly with big sweeping motions. This puts a player off balance, puts the stick outside of the shoulders, and makes the stick hard to recover back to two hands when pivoting. If the defender cannot get two hands on the stick during the pivot, the advantage is to the attacker. The defender, without two hands on the stick, is usually left flailing with the free hand while getting beaten, or will incur a holding penalty by using the free arm to stop the attacker. The correct stick position should have the stick placed in front of you, slightly outside the right or left shoulder based on the way the offensive player shoots. The stick should only be used with small controlled movements. To clarify, if the player is defending a right handed shooting attacker, then the stick (no matter which way the defender shoots) should have the blade of the stick in front of defender's left shoulder. An offensive player's strength is to the forehand, and so this is the preferred direction to go around a defender. The defender should get the stick in the intended path of the player and wait them out. This will force the offensive player to try to beat the defender on their backhand. This is generally their weakest way of shooting. Players should pivot from backward to forward, while placing two hands on the stick ready to battle "stick on stick". **Fifth-the body-** As the puck is dislodged, or the offensive player's head goes down, the defender can now use the body to separate the player from the puck with the body check (using proper angling as discussed in the body checking segment). He should not jump forward at the player to make a hit, as the defender is now fully committed, having stopped their backward momentum. Should the offensive player avoid the body check, the defender will be badly beaten and make the offense player look like a superstar. The defender should initiate the check while engaging two hands on the stick during the pivot and angling of the offensive player. It is important to get both hands on the stick to improve your strength and to control the offensive player. This will also improve the chances of recovering the puck after the hit. Contact should be made after the attacker has made a move to one side or the other, preferably with the body turning to control the defender's body. "Stick on Stick" gives maximum opportunity to recover the puck. Everyone sees the big hits of the NHL during which the stick is nowhere near the puck. This occurs generally when the defender has caught the offensive player with their head down or looking backward for a pass. It rarely occurs when the player has the puck under control with their head up. Remember to always finish the check even if the puck is released. No matter whether the check is successful or not, the defender must stay with that attacker. The defender should stay with the attacker until their team has recovered the puck, or the back checking players have arrived in the zone.

Forwards are frequently asked to fill in for rushing or pinching defensemen during the game. However, it is rare to see forwards playing defense in practice, especially in a one on one drill. How can we expect the forwards to learn to defend the one on one or recover the puck in their own zone under offensive pressure, if they don't learn the skills in practice? Parents of forwards should be supportive of this training and not resist that their children are being taught the basics of all positions. Many elite club teams and NHL teams employ a forward on the point for power plays. That opportunity will not be afforded to a player who can't skate backward and handle the basics of being a defender. Coaches-- simply cycling the forwards and defense- one time on defense and one time on forward through the drills- will give everyone some experience with alternate positions. This practice will also give all players different perspectives on how difficult the other players' roles are. This type of practice approach can also serve as a morale boost for the team as there are great laughs to be had when the forwards get painted pylon orange, or a forward lays out an attacking defenseman with a great check.

# 16

## Body Checking and Angling

*Never attack directly toward the boards.*
*Angle the puck carrier.*
*Check the front of the player by cutting*
*into their path.*
*Make the hit stick on stick.*
*Pin the puck carrier*
*(for a teammate to recover the puck).*
*Keep your hands, elbows and stick down.*

Body checking can be one of the most exciting plays in hockey, and also one of the most dangerous. Far too often though, very little time in practice or game instruction is focused on giving and taking a body check. I continue to see kids racing directly toward a fixed set of boards with a player chasing them. They seem to be expecting a silly stop sign on the back of their game sweater to somehow protect them. Nothing is going to protect them fully, as accidents do happen. However, by following some basic techniques, a player can play safer hockey. A player should never attack or chase a puck carrier directly toward the boards. The body should be angled, and the player should take a path to the puck which will allow the player to arrive at the puck with their body (shoulder) touching the boards. It is critical that the chasing player take an identical path, as the puck carrier may move, drop or trip.  If the attacker is on a direct path to the boards, this can lead to the attacking player incurring a serious injury by falling over the fallen player, and going head first into the boards.

After ensuring that the attacking player is always approaching the targeted player on an angle, the basic body checking principle is to ensure that the body checker applies the body check with their stick on the same side as the stick of the puck carrier.  "**Stick on Stick**", is the key phrase.  The reason for this is simple, but often missed in our desire to have players inflict the maximum hit on the other player.  Parents, it may seem to be great fun when your child is making the hit, but much less enjoyable when your child is taking the hit.  Body checking is a skill used to regain control of the puck.  When applying a proper body check, the stick and head should be facing the puck in the ideal position to recover the puck if it is freed from the puck carrier.  A body check applied without stick on stick will, in most cases, result in the loose puck being recovered by the puck carrier.  That player will be facing the puck and aware of its location, with their stick closer to it.  At the younger ages, proper instructions, on angling and body position, are critical to safe and fair play.  Emphasize with your child that body checking from behind is never acceptable- no matter what the game score- or no matter what the other player has done.  I would rather see fights than a check from behind.  There are a few coaches who might teach or promote presenting a player's back to attacking players in an attempt to draw penalties. This practice must be stopped to protect the players. Parents should watch the team and your child's actions closely, ensuring that everything about checking is being taught to protect your child. If you notice your child presenting their back intentionally or inadvertently to an opposing player, then address the issue sternly as unacceptable. No game is worth a serious injury.

# 17

## Changing Lines - when to change and when not to.

*Shift length of 45 seconds is ideal.*
*Change when the puck is deep in the opponent's zone.*
*Change when your team is in control of the situation.*
*Keep your eyes on the play at all times,*
*and return to the play on turnovers.*
*Don't change in your own end.*
*Don't change when you are part of the back check.*
*Don't change when the play is near your bench.*

Who wants to change and leave the ice when the puck is moving toward the other team's net? Especially if you might become part of a scoring play. This is the same offensive end of the rink in which you collect points and achieve personal recognition. The "Team comes first" (BP) is not just a saying: it is a belief. This belief must drive the players to change at the correct time of the game, despite how it affects them personally. This is a tough skill to master, and like all other skills, it requires practice time. Players generally don't like changing when on offense. As a result, you will see many players changing on the back check to avoid the hard skate into their zone at the end of a shift. Any old timers' game will demonstrate the desire to strongly avoid back checking by changing players. We spend all game trying to create odd man opportunities (BP), and when players leave the ice at the wrong time it allows the other team space and a player advantage. This space will generally lead to scoring opportunities for the other team. Players must be taught that no matter how tired they are, they are more valuable in position on the ice than leaving their team shorthanded while making a change. Players must recognize that the best situation in which to change is when the puck is furthest away from their net, or in the control of their own team.

Most players are taught that 45 seconds is about the right shift length for the average in-shape player to go at full speed before tiring and losing effectiveness. Therefore, players moving out of their zone, who have been on the ice for 35 seconds or more, should be focused on gaining the center line and getting the puck into the offensive zone. This will allow maximum time to change players. The temptation is large, as you move up the ice, to want to go score a goal, but solid team play must be taught. Unless players are in a rush- of 3 on 2, 2 on 1, or a breakaway- a dump will allow the team to execute a full change. In a case in which you have the odd man advantage, then the rush should be completed. As soon as the rush is completed, the last two into the zone are able to peel off for the change, and the third should leave as soon as the player is no longer pressuring the puck. Forwards must be taught that it is critical to get the puck deep into the zone, thus allowing the defense to change. This is especially true in the second period when it is a long change. Too often, one forward, fresh from a change on the back check, will hit the ice and then once the puck is recovered this player may selfishly try to beat defenders after crossing the red line instead of dumping the puck. This results in a turnover and the defense missing an opportunity to change. This selfish play is about the lack of player awareness and team play (BP). The defense may now be forced to stay on the ice for an additional 30 to 45 seconds, working down low in their end against fresh forwards from the other team. Tired players, trapped in a defensive position for too long, will lead to breakdowns and goals against. Icing the puck (non NHL) or dumping it deep out of the zone may be required in an emergency and should be supported. This action will allow for a change to stop sustained pressure, and will allow tiring defenders to change. Goalies also need to recognize that with tired players on the ice any chance to cover the puck and cause a whistle is greatly appreciated.

Changes should rarely occur on the back check (to your own end between the two blue lines) and not for the first or second back checker if 4 players from the other team are in the rush. The last two back checkers, if they are not critical to the play, can skate past the bench for a chance to change. The player coming on the ice can then leave the bench when the player going off the ice is within 10 feet of the bench. In this situation, you can actually gain ice on a change. In a situation in which the other team dumps and makes a full change, then and only then, should changes while the puck is in our end be made. Changes could be made by all the back checking forwards and potentially one defenseman.

Changes in the neutral area between the two blue lines also should rarely occur. The exception to this would be the winger closest to the bench if your team has control. No team can afford to play a player short in this area during a change, as this advantage invariably leads to the puck going into your zone, and then no one gets to change. Players should stay on the ice and compete for the puck. They can then work to recover the puck and dump the puck in and get a change. There should be no stick handling, or trying to beat players in the neutral area, when you have tired players on the ice. Your teammates, seeing you with control, are counting on you to dump the puck, and any turnover will catch everyone out of position. Work the 10 extra seconds to gain control and dump the puck in for a proper line change. This is always better than leaving out-manned and tired teammates to spend another 45 seconds on the ice.

All players, especially defensemen, must be taught to watch the play at all times (BP) when changing. Players must be instructed, from the earliest ages, that should the play change direction quickly due to a turnover, they are fully supported by the coaching staff to return to the play without changing. Too many times players are called to the bench for a change and turn to the bench, ignoring the play. A turnover might occur behind the player coming to the bench, and the player cannot react, causing a bad change which potentially leads to a goal against. A similar situation often occurs when a player is returning from the penalty box. The player may have been signaled to return to the bench upon leaving the penalty box as their line is not on the ice. This player is often seen skating across the ice ignoring the puck and the play, thus missing their opportunity to play the puck or pick up a defensive responsibility. Each returning penalized player should be instructed to focus on the play before leaving the box, recognize which position is not covered by the players on the ice, and if required, know enough to stay on the ice in that position until a change can be made. As a final point to the returning penalized player, why should it be the responsibility of the coaches, parents, and teammates on the bench to tell the players on the ice that the penalty is over? Any player leaving the box should be communicating (BP) at the top of their lungs that the penalty is over, the team is back to even strength, and which position the player is assuming. For everyone wondering why the goalie of the team with the man advantage is banging their stick on the ice loudly about 5 seconds before the penalty is over, it is to inform their team's defenders to be aware an opposing player entering the ice behind them. Once again this is a key communication (BP) by the goalie that if not made could lead to the returning penalized player coming back on the ice and receiving a breakaway pass. This is a good example of why a goalie must be focused on the game during times when the puck is in the opponents end. Goalies can also bang their stick during the game to alert defenders that an opposing player, due to a change or due to a player leaving the offensive end late, is now in behind the defense unnoticed.

To all parents who volunteer to open a players' door for your team- this is greatly appreciated. It is, however, an important role and can influence the outcome of the game, so the job should not be taken lightly. You must be aware of where the puck is at all times, and only open the door when the area in front of the bench is not in the play, or not soon to be in the play. Just because a player is coming to the bench does not necessarily mean that the door must open. As we all know, each team is only allowed a maximum of 5 skaters on the ice at any time, except if the goalie is pulled. "Too many men on the ice" penalties are coaching errors, and the person working the door is part of the coaching staff. If the play is close to the bench, and you are not sure of making a safe player change, then hold the door closed. Return the player to the action until the play has left the bench area, and a safe time to change is found. The other reason for not opening the door when the play is near the bench is that an open door represents a significant safety risk. A player being checked into an open or partially open door can suffer serious injury. We have all cringed in the stands as the play approaches the bench area. The person working the door sees a player coming to change, completely disregards the proximity of the play, and opens the door, creating a dangerous situation. I have heard too many times from bench staff, "The player was tired and wanted to change. What am I supposed to do?" The action you are supposed to do is put safety first, **<u>DON'T</u>** open the door! Tell the player to continue playing until you are sure the area in front of the bench is clear for a safe player change. The player should not be changing when the play is in front of their bench anyway, so make sure this is discussed when the player eventually leaves the ice. When the time is right to open the door, make sure the player going onto the ice is ready at the door. When the player leaving the ice is about to enter the area 10 feet from the bench (the legal changing area), the door should be opened, and the fresh player should be entering the ice. Players going onto the ice always have priority at the door. If more than one player is changing at the same time, all players entering the ice should be on the ice before the players on the ice attempt to leave. To avoid conflict at the door, older teams will have the players who are going on the ice climb over the boards in the middle of the bench. Those exiting the ice will use the doors. This is not recommended for younger players, as the drop to the ice can lead to an injury. As discussed previously, if the play changes quickly, and if the changing player is not focused on the play, then the parent on the door must communicate verbally with the player to return to the play, reinforced by keeping the door closed. Keeping the door closed is critical, as the player on the ice will finally recognize the emergency situation and return to the play. If the door is open the player who is entering the ice, anticipating the player on the ice changing, will leave the bench and a "too many men on the ice" penalty may ensue. Try to keep the door closed for as long as possible. Only open it when you are 100% sure a change should occur.

# 18

## CLOSE THE GAP

*Defense should keep all opposing players
in front of them.
Keep the space between the defense
and the forwards to a minimum.
Be close to the opposing players closest to your end.
Move up with the play quickly to minimize the gap.*

The strength of any defensive structure is taking away time and space (BP) from the opposition. We discussed how to do this in our end with the 5 man box. We discussed the correct method to use in the offensive zone, correctly fore-checking, with support from all players to close passing lanes, ensuring that a third player is high to back-check and eliminate odd man rushes. So, in the neutral zone how do we ensure that we control time and space? Breaking down a defense involves spreading them out to open up opportunities for the offense to out-man the defenders, and give the offense the advantage. In the neutral zone, if the defensemen do not hustle up the ice and "Close the gap.", or keep the distance between their forwards and themselves to a minimum, then a gap occurs. This gap allows the other team space to pass or skate without resistance. This space also increases the chance of a pass being completed. Once an opponent receives a pass with room, the space allows the player to get up to speed before attacking the defense. The defensemen should be encouraged to move up the ice quickly as the other team's forwards back check, ensuring that they are trailing within 2 stick lengths of the other team's last player. This allows the maximum opportunity to intercept passes, discourage passes, and to angle players before they can get up to speed. An easy break out, caused by too much room given to the opposing forwards, forces your team to have to skate the full length of the ice to recover the puck. Emphasize to your defensemen that this is not a time to rest, and if they are too tired to skate and close the gap, then that indicates a good time to change.

Reducing the gap is critical, but defensemen must give full priority to the opposing players closest to their net, even if they are not the puck carrier. These players are the most dangerous. I would like to use an example to point out the correct player to cover. An opposing player takes the puck from your defensive partner in their zone and starts on a 2 on 1. The player with the puck is at their blue line, and the other forward is at the red line. The player at the red line is the immediate threat. The remaining defending defenseman should be positioned within 1 stick length of the forward at the red line to deter the pass. The player with the puck can skate as much as they want to with the puck, but eventually the lead forward will have to wait at the blue line to avoid going offside. By taking away the pass, the defender gives their team the maximum time to back check in support. Also remember that a player skating with the puck will move slightly slower than without the puck. Force the trailing player to carry the puck, thus increasing the time for support to come. As the offensive players get closer and eventually become equally close to your blue line, then a standard 2 on 1 defense between the two players should be adopted until back checking support arrives. As soon as the support arrives, communicate (BP) which player to take and move quickly to take your player.

Another common situation occurs during a breakout when the opposing winger (in their end) receives the pass on the boards. This player is looking to skate it out, or pass it to his breaking line mates. Some defensemen will remain focused on the puck, staying inside the blue line (with the Parents yelling "Hold the line!" as discussed earlier) and miss the center and winger breaking out of the zone ahead of the puck. The defenseman on the puck side must in this situation, back away from the blue line in front of the centerman. This will take away the easy break out pass to the centerman. The other defenseman will take the other winger, ensuring at worst a 2 on 2, with neither defenseman being trapped in the defensive end. Even if the player with the puck is allowed to skate unimpeded out of the zone because the defense has pulled out, this is preferred. You don't have to hold the line every time. Without back checking support, holding the line may result in giving up an odd man advantage, which is not an option. Hold the line should occur when you are 90% assured of capturing the puck, or taking the man. You have to get one or the other. Staying inside the blue line to take the player is only a viable option when the defenseman has confirmed that the high forward is moving back to cover the breaking forwards. If the high forward is not there, only 100% assurance of getting the puck allows the defenseman to stay inside the blue line. The defenseman making the hit without capturing the puck is no longer a satisfactory option, no matter how hard the hit may be, as a released puck can lead to a 2 on 1.

# 19

## THE LIGHTS OUT DRILL--
## KNOWING WHERE ALL 12 PLAYERS ARE AT ALL TIMES.

*Know where everyone on the ice is at all times.*
*Estimate where they will be in 1 or 2 seconds.*
*Verbally communicate your position.*

This is the most misunderstood and probably the most important part of any sport, especially in the high paced, free flowing game of hockey, in which players can get hit hard at any time. All attention at the younger ages goes directly to the puck. The parents watch the puck, most coaches watch the puck, and even the TV focuses on the puck, but the game is actually won or lost away from the puck. It must be emphasized to your child that to succeed at hockey, players must see the whole ice. To do this their heads are constantly on a swivel, recording where each player and the officiating staff are on the ice. They must also anticipate where everyone will be 1 or 2 seconds from that moment. Just like in chess, anticipating your opponent's next move can only be done if you know where all the men are. Then it is possible to analyze what the next potential move may be.

Play this little game with your child. Ask them what they saw on any given play from the game just played. Most children will only remember what they did and very little of the situation. Understandably, it is hard to remember the exact situation and where everyone on the ice was located for the whole game. Now, using a video tape of the game, move to the game situation on the TV and play the situation through completely. Discuss the situation again and get their feedback. Now, with the use of the video tape, it is possible to show your child what was missed and how the game situation could have been improved if more awareness of the other players had occurred.

For Coaches—there is a practice drill in which the coach asks the kids to stop on the whistle and close their eyes immediately. They then select two players to keep their eyes closed and ask them a question such as, "How far is Bobby your Left Winger from you?" While the players keep their eyes closed they are asked to point to where the other players are standing. This can be a lot of fun for all, as it encourages awareness of everyone's location on the ice. In the dressing room at an off moment, ask the players to all close their eyes immediately. Ask, "Who is sitting two players to your left?" etc. Keep doing this until it becomes normal practice for your players to be aware of where their teammates are at all times.

In hockey some of the best players seem to make amazing passes without appearing to look in that direction. Those players will use verbal communication from a teammate combined with their ability to maintain a mental picture of all players' positions on the ice, and then project where those players will be in the next few seconds. Players should be taught to swivel their heads constantly, taking new pictures as often as possible as a lot of movement happens in a few seconds. A soft pass to an open area, because the passer is aware that the area is clear, allows the puck receiver to adjust and complete the pass. A lack of awareness of where all players are on the ice may result in a difficult or hard pass being attempted in this situation. In this way a good scoring chance could unnecessarily be lost. How many times have you see this in minor hockey? Great passers adjust the speed of the pass and the time to pass based on a complete awareness of the circumstances. Great receivers of the pass, and generally the top goal scorers, use this awareness to find open spaces. They adjust their speed to get to that ideal spot to receive the pass at the right time. It is not luck that the puck lands on their stick at the right time, or that the goal scorer is perfectly positioned to score on a rebound. The great players have a greater awareness of where each player is on the ice. They constantly assess the whole ice and everyone's position on the ice. These great players then react quickly to move to the best position to succeed. Awareness of everyone on the ice may be the most important skill found consistently in all top players.

Awareness of all players on the ice is especially true for goalies. A pass or shot across the crease could force a quick or emergency movement depending on the positioning of the opposition. As goalies must focus on the puck, it is imperative that they know where everyone is, or where they may end up being, in the zone. In this way, the goalie can move out to block a shot knowing whether or not the offensive player by the crease is covered or not. The goalie must also communicate with his defenders on missed defensive assignments, open players, breakout options, or just in helping to protect the defense when offensive players are attacking them from behind. A strong skating goalie can be a significant asset to the defense if the goalie can leave the goal crease and play the puck. It is critical that the goalie be aware of open space and opposing player locations, as a misplayed puck outside the goal crease can be very risky and result in an easy goal against.

For the goalies and the players the general rule is, make your assessments and determine your top options for success before you receive the puck. Be aware of everyone on the ice at all times. Don't start to assess and find options after receiving the puck. The time to think is before you get the puck.

# 20

## ACCEPTABLE BEHAVIOR FROM THE PARENTS.

*Team is always first.*
*Positive support for all players from the stands*
*Positive communication after the game*
*Support your coaching staff*
*and keep bad comments private.*
*Take an active volunteer role to support the team.*
*Parents are responsible for their child's equipment,*
*behavior and attendance.*

Parents, this is a key area of the book. I may surprise you by not asking you to just sit in the stands and clap nicely; this is not a reasonable request. Hockey costs are soaring and being involved puts large demands on your time. As such, you have expectations from your child, the coaches, and for that matter, the referees. As hockey is a life lesson, you have to ask yourselves what lessons you want your child to learn from the game and from their parents. I believe you should look to hockey to offer to your children the following positive developmental opportunities. These opportunities will offer solid stepping stones to success in whatever career your child may chose after school.

1. **Teamwork**. Throughout their lives your children will continually be asked to work with other people

*Hockey For Parents*

in situations in which the Team/Company success is driven by teamwork. Trusting your teammates to be there for you, and being there for them no matter what your comfort zone, are key components of teamwork. These practices contribute greatly to growth as a person. Your child must learn to put aside personal goals, and sometimes feelings, for the benefit of team success.

2. **Communication.** Learning to communicate in a team environment will require dealing with teammates with different upbringings and backgrounds. Quite frankly there will be those you like, and even more importantly those you don't like. Finding the ability to work with everyone for the team good is an important skill, and starts with the parents. Racial or derogatory comments are never acceptable and may be repeated by your child. More importantly, they may influence how your children think and feel about their teammates. If your child hears you putting down teammates, how is your child naturally going to react, even if they feel differently? The key is that comments and after game reviews should focus on the fundamentals and not on personalities. If parents have to talk about individual players, then they should do it privately, not with their children. After a game is a good time to review specific situations privately, but take the emotion out of the discussion if possible. Always start by asking your child what the coaches thought of the game

as a team effort. Then ask if any comments were made directly to your child to get a flavor of the environment your child has just come from. If the coaches have just delivered a stern reprimand, then continuing it in the car will not get you the results you are looking for. If your child has played a strong game, this is the time to point out the key areas and congratulate their play. If the game was not one of their best, first ask yourself, as a parent, a few key questions. Was the whole team out of whack in that game, and no matter what your child did, would it have made a difference? Has your child been sick? Is your child still dealing with an injury that may be affecting stamina or may be causing timid play? The injury may be healed, but the pain that was felt when it occurred is not easily forgotten. Could anything else in their life such as birthdays, holidays, family illnesses etc., be affecting their concentration? With all the outside factors in mind, it is probably better to wait until later in the day, or the following day, to talk about problems. But if you know you child can discuss the game afterward, then focus on the technical (areas to improve) and reemphasize the team system and approach. Don't contradict the coaching staff. Make a note of the points that your child indicates are confusing directions from the coaching staff. If you don't understand the direction being taken by the coach, then ask the coach privately for clarification. Once the clarification has been made, then meet with the player and coach together to go over the clarification. This approach is critical for the player to see the coach and parent working together to deliver a common message. Never make statements to your child such as, "The coach doesn't know what he is talking about" no matter what your true feelings are. If that is your feeling, take your queries to the coach. If the coach completely disagrees with your ideas or understanding of the approach to the game, then what should you do? If it is specific to your child and not team comments, then discuss it and deal with it as you see fit. If they are team system comments, then you have to make the commitment to approach your child with the coach's expectations and be perceived as supporting the coach. Many business managers have to deliver tough messages in the business world. We may not fully support or agree with all of them, but our jobs and futures with that company are based on our ability to deliver our best effort toward achieving the Company/Team goals. Sometimes we all have to admit that there might be another way to get to the same goal. Remember, just like in the work world, any negative feedback that gets back to the coaches can only hurt your child's opportunities.

3. **Communication from the Stands.** Most players, as they get older, begin to tune out the noise from the stands to the point of not hearing a word said. On this basis, yelling to your child from the stands has little effect but to embarrass yourself. The better the coaching staff, the less noise from the

stands has been my experience. Parents generally will defer to the coaching staff if they are confident that the necessary instruction and correction is on-going, and given fairly to all players. Parents seeing deficiencies on the ice that are not being corrected on the bench, have a tendency to become more vocal, in an attempt to give directions that they feel are not being addressed by the coach. I would ask that you take one more step before communicating from the stands. That is to meet with the coaching staff and express your concerns. Use specific situations and find out what the coaching staff is seeing. It is natural that every parent watches their child more than any other player on the ice. When I was coaching I received some of the best feedback from knowledgeable parents who asked that I keep an eye on a certain situation, or that I review directly with their child something discussed at home that the player was confused about. This type of communication should be welcomed by all coaches. When the parents work closely with the coaches the team is then expanding its knowledge base, which can only help in all the players' development. In the situation where it is a tough year and frustrations are brewing, the parents have to remember that it is only one year of a hockey career. Try to project a positive attitude and support your child, as they are probably having a tough year also. If all else fails and you are finding it hard to stay positive, get busy at work or at home. Stay away from the rink because your frustration might lead to a situation you will quickly regret.

4. **<u>Parents in the dressing room.</u>** Some coaches like to keep parents away from the dressing room and away from the team. In fact, they like it better if there is no communication with the parents at all. Some coaches have stated that conversations with parents are usually bad conversations, as few parents want to see them with good news. These coaches claim that if the parents are not complaining, then they are just trying to get their kids more ice time. I see parents as a critical part of the team. It is in the best interest of the coaching staff to have all the parents as informed as their players. The parents should understand the expectations of the coaches and also the "System" they are going to play. Parents can't support the coaches if they don't know what is being taught and only get the information from their young child. Publishing and discussing team rules is the first necessary communication to ensure understanding of the critical issues of arrival times, dress requirements etc. A playbook or team systems book handed out to all players and parents is critical to teaching all the team expectations. It is also much easier for parents to support the coach's initiative when they know what the initiative is. Include the parents in the team meetings when the playbook is reviewed, and welcome the parents' involvement and questions. A progress report every month on the goals for next month, and

success with last month's goals, is also critical to ensure that everyone is on the same page. The best way to show progress is to utilize videotape of games, from the beginning and each month, as support for the monthly report. They make great keepsakes, and most parents, when they go back a few tapes, will realize just how much progress the team has made.

5. **Most Teams now have a Team Parent.** This role was established to have someone who can communicate for the parents in cases in which parents are not comfortable talking directly with the coaches. This can be an effective way to get feedback and ask questions, but I still recommend that the parent talk directly with the coaching staff and hear the answers given first hand.

6. **Support the Manager of the team.** The parents, along with the team manager, must take full responsibility for team functions and administration. Keep this away from the coaching staff. Most coaches are volunteering their time, and as such, have enough time invested in being at the rink and preparing for all games and practices. They should not need to worry about anything other than coaching. Always remember that all decisions must still be approved by the head coach before being implemented.

7. **A parent's responsibility.** Parents are responsible for the players' equipment, skate sharpening,

taping of sticks and for relating to the trainer all health and life issues that may affect their children. Communicate, and give the coaches the best opportunity to make hockey a positive event for your child. If you have little hockey experience and you just need help, then no problem- just ask.

8. **Overused phrases.** The statements, "The kids are just having fun." or, "They are only here to have fun." are the most overused phrases I hear in hockey. They are used by parents mainly as an excuse for something. Having fun is a result of hard work and good team work, both conducted in a positive and safe environment. Fun also has to be had by all players on the team. One strong player may have fun, hogging the puck, stick handling through the other team, and scoring multiple goals, but are their teammates really having fun? Probably not. The fun should start as soon as players walk into the arena, but the coaching staff does not become your child's babysitter. The coaches are under strict regulations and scrutiny, and dealing with an insubordinate child is probably the hardest task for a coach. Don't the coaches also deserve to have fun? I believe fun starts with respect, and respect for adults and authority starts at home. A child hanging off the rafters, swearing, or otherwise misbehaving in the rink before a game or practice, should be dealt with by the parents not the coaching staff. These actions may be "fun" for your children, but are not appropriate for a hockey team, as they

are representing their team and centre. A child may be injured, or cause injury to others, which by itself is not good. It could also cause the team to lose a valuable player. More importantly, every rink has rules that are made to reduce insurance costs, to make it financially manageable to even have organized hockey. You may not like the rules, just as you may not agree with some of the rules at work, but it is not acceptable to change them to fit your individual tastes. The coaches will set rules, but the coaches need parental support even if you may personally feel differently. Remember this is a team (parents, players and coaches) so your support is expected. As we go back to hockey reflecting life, respecting other peoples' property and rules is a key life lesson. As a last note on respect. I blame society for this one, but as we get closer to being friends with our kids, we sometimes lose focus on the point that a coach deserves the respect of the position. Therefore every time I hear, "Hey Mark, throw me some tape." my back goes up. On my team no response would be given. The coach is referred to as Coach (First name), or Mr. (last name), without exception. Proper manners, which include please and thank you, are also mandatory. They are not to be ignored just because we are having fun. Ultimately, my experience is that players have the most fun when they play for teams with strong discipline (applied equally to all, including coaches) and a focus on team success. Surprisingly enough, most of these teams are winning teams. I wonder if this is a coincidence.

9. **<u>Winning in not a goal; it is a result.</u>** What does this mean? Of course we play all games to win, or they wouldn't keep score and hand out awards, but I often ask parents and coaches whether winning is really the most important goal. Should we be willing to take away the fun, and the life lessons to be learned from the game, for the sole purpose of winning a $10 trophy at the end of the year? I hope everyone's answer is no. Is it worth winning if everyone on the team is not having fun? I see so many top level hockey teams on which the staff cuts their bench back in the first and second period. They run the same power play and penalty kill units from the beginning to the end of the season. This practice only rewards a select few kids with extra ice time and does not develop the entire team. I also hear idle chatter from the stands, "Why is that player on the ice?", or "Doesn't the coach want to win?" If a player was good enough to make the team, then that player should be good enough to learn to play all facets of the game. The only way to do that is to expose all players to all facets in practice and then in games. I will agree that should a player miss practice time, and not learn the coaches' expectations, then game opportunities will be sacrificed. That player cannot be expected to perform, and should not expect to hold back the other 4 skaters on the ice due to their lack

of knowledge. The key is that all kids should be expected to perform, and should be given practice time for all specialty team situations. Parents, it is equally important to study with your child just like school. The play books handed out by the coaches at the beginning of the year are to be studied and reviewed so that mentally the child is prepared to perform. Parents- in the last few minutes of a game, a key situation late in the season or playoffs, or in a tournament- the coaches must reserve the right to select the top players. The choice of these players may change based on current game performance. This decision on who to play could extend or win a game, and may move the team on in the playoffs or in a tournament. That result will mean that the whole team will get more ice time. My experience with players convinces me that they know who should be on the ice at critical times, and they have no issues with stepping aside for the benefit of the team. The players especially appreciate any coach who asks them to step aside at some crucial point as long as the players know that in the next few games, should the score dictate, they will be given extra opportunity to develop. They may be asked to come back, and start the next game, and basically be reassured that they are a crucial part of the team and that they will be rewarded for putting the team first. The last note on why winning is a result not a goal. A team of players working together in a "System" all equally treated and developed, will prove a formidable foe for any team that makes a habit of shortening their bench early in the game. The full bench will eventually wear down the short bench in 2 game-a-day tournaments or in back to back playoff match ups. I can only look to experience to say that teams using all their players are much more successful, are having more fun, and have the fewest parental issues and concerns. A strong team effort is FUN.

10. **<u>Research your coaches before committing.</u>** As a parent it is critical to do your research on the coaching staff before tryouts and well before you commit your child to the team. It is important to understand the coaches' philosophies and objectives for the year. Coaches usually don't communicate with the parents until after tryouts, and then it is generally too late, as your child has already been selected for the team. For most coaches, it is not their first year coaching, so find out where they coached previously. If this is locally, contact parents from previous teams and get their feedback. Get feedback, if you can, from a parent of a top 5 player and a bottom 5 player, to see if the experience for both is consistent. Every parent must try to evaluate their child honestly during tryouts, and getting feedback from someone outside of the team, if possible, is ideal. Get someone to watch a tryout if you have concerns, preferably someone who has seen last year's team play and can tell you honestly where your child fits on the team. If you evaluate your child in the last 2 defensemen, or as a

third line forward, then the coaching philosophy is critical to your decision whether or not your child will play on that team. You had better know the philosophy before you sign a card. A coach who will shorten the bench and is focused on his few top players will not help your third line forward grow and develop. Wearing the team jacket, or being able to say that your child plays top level hockey, should have no bearing on your decision. It is not about the parent; it is about what is best for your child. It may be better to play for a weaker team if you disagree with the philosophy on the stronger team. This may offer your child ice time equal to the other players and a chance to learn and play on specialty teams, which would be better than sitting on the bench of the better team. If it truly is about fun, then make sure you put your child on a team on which they will have fun. Lastly, if you evaluate your child in the bottom 5 on the team, and your research indicates that the coach has a history of fair play and of developing all their players, then take this opportunity and accept the card as offered. Your child may sacrifice some ice time in the last 5 minutes of a crucial game, but if your child continues to progress, does additional work outside the team on power skating, shooting or whatever is their weakness, they will improve. Other opportunities, from suspensions or injuries, may give your child a chance to prove themselves capable. Your child will generally learn more with a good coach, playing at the highest level possible, and practicing and playing against the best. Each level of hockey is significantly faster, more physical, and more mentally demanding. This competition is necessary for your child's development, but not at the sacrifice of significant ice time.

11. **<u>Is hockey worth all the effort?</u>** Parents, at the end of every year, we all walk away definitely financially poorer, tired of all the running around, fundraising, and bad diet meals eaten on the run. If we are lucky our child gets a $10 trophy. At this point the child may ask if he can go to a friend's house to play, seemingly without appreciating all your time and effort. Why? Because they just want to play, be with their friends and have some fun. The biggest success of any year, the only one I evaluate the year on as a coach, is when the player shakes your hand, says thank you and states that they are looking forward to playing hockey next year. If your child has enjoyed the experience enough to want to play the following year, then the year has been a success. Remember that kids have a lot of outside pressures from friends and schoolmates. With idle time, these influences can sometimes lead them astray. Being involved in organized sports keep your child active, healthy and in a situation in which you know where they are and what they are doing. This involvement in sports will help your child's character development and may change the direction your child takes in life. Athletes and former athletes are highly successful, and they are

highly recruited in the business world because of the lessons learned playing competitive team sports. So my recommendation is to do everything you can as a parent to keep your child having fun in hockey. Put them in the right situations so that they stay in hockey. After they finish their playing careers, your child may take up refereeing or even coaching, and hopefully give back some of their time to the younger players. Maintaining involvement in hockey is far more important than winning, or the prestige of being on the best team.

# 21

## PULLING THE GOALIE

*There is no right time to do it.*
*Be aggressive as a goal against*
*doesn't change the result.*

Pulling the goalie is arguably one of the most exciting times in a hockey game. The trailing team pulls out all the stops to try to tie the game. It is also the time when the parents for the leading team get their loudest, yelling to the kids that the net is empty. Why do this? There is not a need to score at this point. The only reason to yell, "The net is empty!" is to have their child score an easy goal, selfishly trying to improve their personal stats. As the theme of this book is team play, I don't understand why a team with a one goal lead needs this information. They do not need to score again to win, and are trying desperately to get the puck out of their end to relieve the pressure as they play against 6 attacking skaters. The biggest mistake that can be made in this situation is that a player, on their own side of center ice, attempts to take a shot at the net trying to score. The player may miss, causing an icing call and a resulting face-off in their own end. The unselfish team-play would be to dump the puck off the boards, thus avoiding an icing into the other team's zone. The respect that this type of player will receive from the coaching staff and from teammates should be far more positive than scoring the goal. Good coaches should reward that player with extra ice time the next time their team is in the lead late in the game. That player has shown an ability to put the team's interests first. If the player is over center ice, and the path to the net is clear, a shot should be taken, as a goal will help clinch the game. Remember though, that if the path to the net is not clear and there is a risk of losing the puck, then it is still better team play to drive the puck into the zone or shoot the puck into the corner. This uses up as much time as possible.

Watch an amateur or professional hockey game with one team down by one goal. Crowd anticipation grows, as they wait to see the goalie pulled for the extra attacker (skater), and the clock gets closer to 1 minute remaining. Do you ever ask yourself why teams wait for the clock to hit the 1 minute mark before starting to call the goalie to the bench? A solid reason is that 1 minute is the maximum time the 6 skaters on ice can perform at top efficiency without changing. A change is not practical during the time the goalie is pulled, as this will open ice, and might allow the other team the opportunity to gain control and get over center for an easy scoring opportunity. But is there a hockey rule I missed that says you are not allowed to pull the goalie prior to the 1 minute mark? I know there is not. There are, however, a few times when you might pull the goalie earlier than the one minute mark.

One example might occur with 90 seconds or less to go when your team might have a face-off in the defending team's zone. This is an ideal time to start with 6 players inside the zone, as it will allow you to outnumber the other team no matter where the puck goes on the draw. As the offensive team has the extra man, the offense must have one extra player on the puck until gaining control. If the defenders have 2, the offense must have 3. If the closest person to make the third is the defenseman on the blue line then the defenseman should enter the battle for the puck. If the defenders have 3 then the offense has 4. It is so bothersome to watch minor hockey when the goalie is pulled, and we then see 3 players standing in front of the net and one lonely player battling 2 and 3 defending players for the puck. At this point many in the stands are yelling that their child is open in front of the net, and that the puck should be passed in front. As it only takes one person to score, it would be wiser to have 2 of the players from in front of the net go to help get the puck. Parents yelling, "Help out!", "Two men on the Puck!" or anything similar would be more appropriate and more helpful.

In the last 5 minutes of the game, if your team is down by 2 or more goals and the other team is 1 or 2 players short due to penalties, then this may be the time to apply extra pressure and pull the goalie. I have seen this work effectively. After scoring the first goal using this strategy, the team that has scored (with the goalie now returned to the net) has the momentum to come out strong and score again. The leading team is now under greater pressure and pressure leads to mistakes.

Don't miss this type of opportunity by waiting for the last minute to pull the goalie.

We discussed earlier that hockey has similarities to chess and that coaches can, by their decisions, change outcomes of games positively or negatively. Good coaches making good decisions and adjustments are worth 1 goal a game over the length of a season. So with 2 to 3 minutes to go, the coaching staff may catch the other coach holding back his best defenders for the final minute. A quick pull of the goalie before the one minute mark, with your best offensive unit on the ice, may catch the other coach with the wrong players on the ice. I look at it this way. The team, in this situation, has gone a full game and they are down by one goal. If they can get their best plus an extra player against the other team's second unit for one minute, this has to be better than best versus best for the last minute or less. This can become more evident when, at the end of a game the coaches can't get the goalie to the bench due to pressure in their end. This early pull of the goalie is even more advantageous if you are playing against a team that has only been coached to use top players in special team situations. If their top players are caught on the bench, this leaves players who are not accustomed to playing in this situation on the ice. Hopefully your coach will have taught every player on your team to play in all situations. In that case coaches will not be able to use this strategy against your team.

# 22

## DROPPED YOUR STICK? THEN PICK IT UP!

*Complete the initial play.*
*Pick up your stick or get off the ice.*
*Communicate the situation to all your players and adjust.*

This is a small chapter I felt necessary to include. Sometimes you see hockey players skating all around the ice without a hockey stick. The players are trying to be like their TV heroes-- blocking shots, remaining in coverage, and doing whatever is necessary to stay in the play. But what can they really accomplish without a hockey stick? With the new crackdown on holding, and with other penalty offenses, a player playing without a stick is just looking for a penalty, as the players' first response is to use their hands to grab. This will result in a penalty, and the team will then be short handed for 2 minutes, or less if the other team scores. My thoughts on this are simple. Picking up a stick takes the player out of the play for a maximum of 10 seconds, not the 2 minutes received for a penalty. I recommend that a player complete the initial play when the stick is lost. By then, teammates realizing there is a player without a stick, can move to a defensive penalty kill position for the 10 seconds or less it takes the player to get a stick and get back into position. Once the stick is recovered, the player communicates the fact to the team that they are back in the play, and then normal positions can be resumed. Playing 20 seconds or more without a stick, which I see on a regular basis, is like giving the other team a free powerplay. The player should complete the initial play, and when no longer pressuring the puck carrier then the player should **<u>GET THE STICK.</u>** If the stick is broken, once the initial play is over that resulted in the stick breaking, the players should communicate with their teammates and get to the bench. The player will either change (usually the best as you can take advantage of the 10 foot rule) or get a new stick and return to the play. The player should not stay out on the ice without a stick.

There are times when defensemen might have a broken stick while playing in their own end. Often the forwards all rush to pass their sticks to the defenseman who has broken their stick. This is done because the forwards see that the defenseman's role is closer to the net and it is viewed as more critical that the defenseman have a stick. I agree fully that their role is more critical in front of the net; however it may result in a 6'6" defenseman playing with a 5'9" player's stick and/or a wrong-handed one. Therefore the team has 1 player playing without a stick and 1 playing with the equivalent of half a stick. Your defensive strength becomes even weaker, not stronger, which was the purpose of passing the stick. If forwards are taught to play the basic defenseman positions, then why would the forward and defenseman not switch positions? This puts a defender in front of their net with full equipment (their own stick) and puts the player without a stick closer to their bench. When the communication is made amongst all the defenders, the defenseman without a stick leaves for the bench and changes, or returns with a new stick.

Coaches, this is easily simulated in practice. As you are conducting power play offensive zone drills, move into the drill and grab one of the player's sticks. Throw it into the corner, or announce that it is broken. The defenders now must communicate and move to defensive positions that allow the player without the puck to recover their stick or leave the ice. Defenders should hold the puck on the boards, dump the puck out of the zone, or even ice the puck, to allow the player to change or recover their stick. Some readers may be thinking that if a player leaves to get a stick, this gives the offensive team some big advantage. On 2 minute power plays in the NHL, top teams are lucky to have a 20% success rate. When a player plays without a stick, the team is effectively short handed immediately. If players can quickly communicate and take up their short handed positions, then the 10 seconds or less it takes to get a stick is minimal risk.

# 23

## WHY DO OFFICIALS KEEP BLOWING THEIR WHISTLES?

*Offside*
*Icing*
*Center removed from the face-off*
*The hand pass*
*High Stick touches the puck*
*Playing with a broken stick*
*Puck goes over the glass*
*Goal called back for kicking or gloving it into the net*
*A player is hurt*
*Delayed penalties*
*Too many men on the ice penalty*
*What causes a penalty shot?*
*How do you know what the penalty is for?*

**Offside.** The puck must go over the opposition's blue line before your players can enter the zone. The other skaters must have contact with the blue line, or be outside the blue line, to remain onside as the puck enters the zone. The key point is that it is not a straight line upwards from the blue line (as in crossing the goal line in football) so if a player lifts their back foot off the ice, and has their other foot inside the blue line, the play will be called offside. The feet placement is the key, so that a player lying on the ice with his feet inside the zone, body on the line, and head outside, is still offside. In Canada, a player is allowed to shoot the puck into the zone when other players are over the blue line (a delayed offside is signaled by the official putting their hand straight up over their head). As long as no one on the offensive team touches the puck, the play continues. If all offensive players get outside the zone at the same time (one at a time is not sufficient) then the delay will be removed by the official dropping their hand. The players can then enter the zone and play the puck. Should the offensive team touch the puck during a delayed offside, then the whistle is blown and the face-off is on the dot outside the offensive zone. An exception is made if the offensive team is aware of the offside and does not attempt to clear the zone immediately, or if an offense player touches the puck on purpose in the zone. The official can, at their discretion, call for the face-off to be all the way back in the defensive zone (an intentional offside). In areas of the USA automatic offside rules apply, which means that the whistle is blown immediately when the official determines an offside has occurred. Touching the puck in the offensive zone is not required. Intentionally shooting the puck back into the offensive zone causing an offside can result in the face-off coming back to the defensive zone (an intentional offside).

**Icing.** Occurs when a player shoots the puck from their side of center ice (on the center line is not icing) and the puck clears the red goal line fully. A shot that hits the goal is not icing. The old rule was that the icing was waved off if the puck went through the crease. This no longer applies. Icing can also be waved off by an official if the defender had a reasonable chance of playing the puck, or if the official determines that the player let up skating after a slow moving puck. Another possible controversial call occurs when a puck goes past a defensive player hard in the air. An official can rule that the defender did not have a reasonable chance of playing the puck; therefore the official will still call icing. No player is assumed to be able to pick the puck out of the air with their stick, so parents take it easy on the official on close calls. If the puck touches any opposition player's body or stick while in its path toward icing, the icing call should be waved off. A puck touched by a teammate before the center line does not negate the icing. If icing is called, the face-off will be in the defensive end of the team causing the icing.

**Center removed from the face-off.** This occurs when the official determines that the center is not lining up correctly for the face-off. Correct alignment would mean that their stick must be on the ice at the bottom of the face-off dot and their feet squared up to dot. It can also occur if another player encroaches inside the circle before the puck is dropped, or a player or their stick moves past the hash marks (lines at sides of the circle that are there to show the separation that the players must maintain until the puck is dropped). If another player causes the center to be removed from the face-off, this player cannot then take the face-off. To speed up play the official will blow their whistle to signal play is about to commence and they are ready to drop the puck. If one team, given reasonable time to get ready, is not in position when the whistle blows, that center should be removed from the face-off. Any further delays may lead to a 2 minute delay-of-game penalty against that team.

**Hand-Pass**. A hand-pass, or hitting the puck with your hand or arm, directly to a player on your own team in your own end (inside your blue line) is a legal pass, and play continues. A hand-pass outside of your blue line directly to a teammate (not touched first by the player making the hand-pass or the other team) is whistled down, and the face-off takes place at the closest dot. If the hand-pass occurs inside the offensive zone, the resulting face-off will be held outside the offensive zone blue line. The play with the most controversy is a hand-pass that is made inside your blue line and is touched first by another player on your team outside the blue line. This is whistled by the officials as a hand-pass, as the first touch after the hand pass did not occur inside your blue-line. The face-off will be brought back to the dot in your zone.

**A high stick touching the puck**. Any time players make contact with the puck by lifting their sticks above the height of their shoulders for younger players, or above the height of the net for older players, the other team must touch the puck first for the play to continue. If the player or a teammate touches the puck, the play is stopped and a face-off occurs. That face-off is at the dot closest to your end from the point at which it was touched or outside the offensive zone if the high stick occurred in the offensive zone.

**Playing with a broken stick.** A player who breaks their stick must immediately drop the broken stick. The player can continue to play without the stick, return to the bench and change, or be passed a new stick from anyone on the bench and then return to the play. Continuing to play, or just carrying the stick after you realize it is broken, will result in a 2 minute penalty. The goalie can continue to play with a broken stick until the whistle is blown, at which point a new stick can be brought to the goalie. Remember, the goalie cannot leave the goal area during a stoppage without the approval of the official, and in an obscure rule, should the goalie leave the net during a stoppage without permission of the official, the official can insist the goalie be replaced by the back up goalie. The goalie can return to the ice at the next whistle, or while the game is in process, if the coach so chooses.

**Goalie loses their stick.** A skater can pass their stick to the goalie to ensure that the goalie has a stick. While the play continues, a player can pick up the loose goalie's stick and pass it to the goalie. During the time the player has the goalie stick in hand any attempt by the player to participate in the play will result in a 2 minute penalty for playing with two sticks. The player does not have to touch the puck for the penalty to be called. Intentionally skating in front of the puck carrier or defending a player away from the puck is sufficient for the penalty to be called. A shot fired at the net that inadvertently hits the player carrying two sticks should not result in a penalty if no attempt was made to stop the puck. Caution should always be taken when carrying the goalie's stick.

**A puck goes over the glass**. If the puck leaves the ice surface, the face-off will be the closest dot to the spot at which the shot was taken. In the offensive zone, if the puck goes directly out or off an offensive player, the face-off will be outside the blue line. If the puck goes off a defender, goalie, or off the net, it will be at a dot in the offensive zone. In high levels of hockey, a puck shot over the glass- if it has not been deflected by a defender in their zone- will result in a 2 minute minor penalty for delay of game. If the goalie sends the puck over the glass, it is an automatic 2 minute penalty. In minor hockey, it is not an automatic penalty if a skater shoots the puck over the glass. A penalty will only be called if it is determined by the referee to be intentional.

**Puck kicked or gloved into the net**. A puck kicked by a skate, thrown, or pushed into the net by a glove will not be allowed as a goal. The face-off will then be brought outside the blue line. A puck that goes into the net after being deflected off a player (including the skate and glove) where there was no intention of propelling it toward the net, is a good goal.

**An offensive player in the crease**. A player is allowed to move through the crease as long as the goalie is not interfered with. Any offensive player can enter the crease area to play the puck after the puck enters the crease area. A goal will be disallowed if an offensive player has at least one foot in the crease prior to the puck going into the net. The official may determine that the player in the crease had no effect on the play. In this case the referee will still allow the goal, but this is the official's call. If the player in the crease also interferes with the goalie prior to the goal, then the goal will be disallowed and a minor penalty for goalie interference should be assessed to the offending player.

**A player is hurt**. This always has the parents yelling at the official, demanding that the official blow the whistle because a player is hurt. Why doesn't that cruel official blow the whistle immediately and get help to the player they howl? The official is responsible for stopping the play immediately only if a serious injury has occurred, or when the team with the injured player gains control of the puck. The reason for this is that many younger players are seen by the official to fall over, but they do not appear to be seriously hurt. If the whistle was blown immediately, a breakaway or scoring chance could be stopped for the opposing team. At the older ages, a crafty player may fake an injury to stop an odd man advantage. If they suspect serious injury, the referees will blow their whistle immediately.

**Delayed penalties**. The official will raise their hand straight above their head when a penalty is to be called. The whistle will not be blown until the team to be penalized gains control of the puck. A deflection or shot on goal not controlled by the goalie will remain in play until control is achieved. The team with the puck can pull the goalie from their net, as the other team cannot score unless a player from the team with the puck somehow scores on themselves. The goalie must be within 10 feet of the bench when the extra skater is sent out. If the player entering the ice leaves the player bench early, the play is immediately stopped and the face-off will be held at center ice, with the original delayed penalty being assessed. Leaving early on a goalie change is not a minor penalty. It causes the play to be stopped and the advantage of playing with the extra attacker is lost. These rules also apply at the end of the game when a team pulls the goalie for an extra attacker. If a goal is scored during a delayed penalty being called against a team already shorthanded, the player in the box will be returned to the ice. The delayed penalty will then be assessed to the offending player for the full 2 minutes. A goal scored during a delayed penalty while both teams are at even strength, results in the penalty being recorded, but the offending player does not have to go to the penalty box as the goal wipes out the penalty.

**Too many men on the ice**. This penalty is assessed if a team has more players on the ice than allowed. In a 5 on 5 situation one team that is playing with 6 skaters and the goalie has too many on the ice. Because players are allowed to enter the ice surface as soon as the players they are replacing get within 10 feet of the bench, the hardest part for coaches and fans to understand is what criteria the official uses to determine when to call a penalty. Some teams will also stretch the 10 foot rule making the call even more difficult. They may receive only verbal warnings from the officials for stretching the 10 foot rule when the play is far away from the bench. When the play is near the bench, or the puck is going through the area in front of the bench, the general rule is that the player entering the ice cannot play the puck before the player they are replacing has stepped completely off the ice. Therefore, if the player entering the ice allows the puck to go past and does not attempt to play it, this would not require a penalty for too many men on the ice. If a player leaving the ice stops and plays the puck when their replacement has already entered the ice, then a penalty for too many men on the ice should be assessed. If the other team sees a change occurring and fires the puck at the bench hitting a player coming on or off the ice inadvertently, this should not be called a penalty. The exception would be if a player purposely plays the puck with the player they are replacing still on the ice. Parents before you begin to yell, "Too many men! Too many men!" remember that the key is that the player must purposely play the puck while the player they are replacing (or being replaced by) is on the ice. If a "Too many men!" penalty is called, it must be served by someone who was on the ice at the time the penalty was called. As this is a delayed penalty, some players may change during the play, but the players on the ice at the time of the call are the only players who can serve the penalty. A player from the bench cannot be substituted to serve the penalty. On a last note, especially with inexperienced officials, the puck may be dropped with one team mistakenly having 6 skaters on the ice. The crowd will immediately start to yell, "Too many men!" to get the referees' attention. This may be understandable, but it is **NOT** a penalty. The game was started with too many men due to an official's error. The whistle should be blown, the clock should be reset if near the end of the game, and the face-off goes back to where the original face-off occurred. This procedure should be followed no matter how long it takes the official to notice it. In effect everything starts over again with no penalty assessed.

**The penalty shot**. For some this is the most exciting play in hockey. As such, the official must be sure, before calling for a penalty shot, that a clear scoring opportunity has been missed due to the incurrence of a penalty by the defending team. The most frequently called penalty shot occurs when one player is on a breakaway. If a defender from behind the puck carrier trips or hooks the player, thus removing a scoring opportunity, then a penalty shot should be called. The official has the tough responsibility of determining if the puck carrier had a clear path to the net, and whether or not the opportunity was lost due to the penalty infraction. Only if this positive determination is made will a penalty shot be called as opposed to a regular two minute penalty. A penalty shot can also be called if a defender puts their hand on the puck, or covers the puck in the crease area of their net. A penalty shot can also be assessed if a stick is intentionally thrown by a defender, in the defensive zone, in an attempt to stop the progress of the attacking team. A penalty shot could also be assessed if, in the last two minutes of the game, a player dislodges their own net intentionally, or a team makes a deliberate illegal substitution. An illegal substitution can be a team sending a player onto the ice away ahead of the player coming off the ice with the intent of stopping a rush or breakaway. In all cases the penalty shot is instead of the penalty being served.

# 24

# Penalties and How To Deal with Multiple Calls on the Same Play

***C.R.A.P.***
***C**ancel as many penalties as possible.*
***R**educe the number of penalties
that cause the teams to play short.*
***A**void taking additional players off the ice
to serve other players' penalties.*
***P**enalties are cancelled in the order they occur.*
*The team has to be shorthanded to get
a player returned (minor only).*
*Offsetting penalties- offending player is off for the
whole penalty time plus a whistle.*
*Short handed goals have no effect on penalties.*

I decided to utilize the C.R.A.P. acronym as an easy to remember saying often heard in the stands by the parent of the penalized player. Thanks to those parents the referees will never forget how to deal with multiple penalty calls. There are so many Minor (2 minute) or Major (5 minute) penalties that I recommend you review your hockey association rules to familiarize yourself with them. A major penalty is usually issued when the penalty leads to a serious injury, or the intent was to cause serious injury. I have included a few pages of examples of how penalties are offset, and who plays short. These processes can be complicated, and they can cause a lot of discussion in the stands and on the bench. The first point is that, on a minor penalty, a goal scored by the team with the player advantage will result in the penalized team having the player returned to the ice. If the team is two players short, the player with the least amount of time remaining to be served will be returned to the ice. The penalized team will then play 1 player short. There could also be a situation in which two penalties are in play, one of which is a major penalty. The player (or player serving their penalty, as a 5 minute major usually comes with a game misconduct in minor hockey) does not return to the ice when a goal is scored, and must serve the full 5 minutes. If a major and minor penalty are being served (to two different players so that the penalized team is playing 3 against 5) even if the major penalty had been called first- a goal against the penalized team will have the minor penalty wiped out. The basic rule is that the shorthanded team, if scored upon, will have a minor penalty removed (offsetting penalties are never affected). In a case in which one player gets a 5 minute major and additional minor penalties that are not offset by the other team's minor penalties, the player will serve the major before the minor penalties. So as an example, if the other team scores in the first 5 minutes of say 9 minutes in penalties (one major and two minor penalties) then no time will be removed from the clock. After 5 minutes a goal will wipe out the remaining time of the 2 minute penalty in progress. The next big issue occurs when both teams have one penalty each. Whether they are major or minor penalties is not important. If a goal is scored, then no one comes out of the penalty box. The key point is that a player is only returned to the ice when an odd man advantage is in place at the time of the goal. In a 4 on 4, or 3 on 3 situation, although both teams are shorthanded, it is not considered an odd man advantage, so all penalties continue, with no change to the times to be served.

**a.** Cancel as many penalties as possible.

This means that if two players, one from each team, go off at the same time with a 2 minute minor penalty, then the penalties offset each other, and neither team plays short. If more penalties are called at the same stoppage, the referee will continue to cancel equal time penalties to minimize the amount of time each team plays shorthanded.

**b.** Reduce the number of penalties that cause the teams to play the least players short.

When reviewing the penalties called, the official will continue to offset penalties to commence play with the fewest players short on either team.

**c.** Avoid taking additional players off the ice to serve other player's penalties.

When players from both teams incur penalties on the same stoppage of play, the penalties will be offset to avoid taking additional players off the ice if possible. Remember that the player assessed, (for example 6 minutes in penalties) with an opposing player getting 4 minutes, must stay in the box for the full 6 minutes, and the other player the full 4 minutes, no matter what goals are scored. The team with 6 minutes must add a player to the penalty box to serve the additional 2 minutes assessed. This team will be shorthanded effective at the drop of the puck. The length of the penalty served, by the player added to the penalty box, will be 2 minutes or shorter if a goal is scored against their team. The player added to the penalty box will return to the ice upon completion of the two minute penalty. Even if a goal is scored, the players serving 6 and 4 minutes respectively must stay in the box until the first whistle after their time is served, with no reduction in time for the goal being scored.

**d. P**enalties are cancelled in the order they occur.

The penalties are announced by the referee and documented on the game sheet. With multiple penalties in which equal time is assessed, the penalties are cancelled in the order in which they were recorded on the game sheet. This is the fairest method for choosing which player's penalty is offset first.

Last note on penalties, this C.R.A.P. method is applied at each stoppage in play. It is not carried over or back to any other penalties called. So if a team is one player short, and 1 second later the other team gets called for a penalty, then both teams play 4 on 4 until the penalties expire. Remember also that on offsetting penalties, the teams do not play short. This means that when the penalized player's 2 minutes or more are over, the penalized players cannot return to the ice until there is a stoppage in play. Also, because they are offsetting, neither team is short, therefore there is no reduction on their penalty time if either team scores. If your team gets 6 off-setting minutes, your players are there for the full 6 minutes, and must wait for the next stoppage of play to return to the ice. This will definitely increase their stay in the box past 6 minutes. Offsetting penalties are not shown on the clock so coaches must make a mental note of the time their players are to return to the ice or they will be constantly asking the referee.

## **Examples of Offsetting Penalties**

| **Team A** | **Team B** | **Player Advantage (pp is power play)** |
|---|---|---|
| 1. 2 min. high stick- #14 | 2 min roughing- #7 | 5 on 5 |

If a goal is scored during the penalties, no one returns as no one is short handed.

Players can only return to ice on first stoppage after 2 minutes served.

| | | |
|---|---|---|
| 2. 2 min. holding - #3 | 2 min roughing - #12 | #3 and #12 offset |
| 2 min. roughing -#7 | | Team B pp 5 on 4 for 2 min. |

Player #3 and player #12 must wait for first whistle after 2 min. served.

If a goal is scored by Team B then the penalty to Team A ends -#7 returns.

| | | |
|---|---|---|
| 3. 2 min. holding - #3 | 2 min roughing - #12 | #3 and #12 offset 2 min. |
| 2 min. roughing -#3 (served by #8) | | Team B pp 5 on 4 for 2 min. |

Player #3 must stay in box for 4 min., #12 for 2 min. no matter if goal is scored by either team. The players would return on a whistle after their time is served. Player #8 picked by the coach from the players on the ice when the penalty was called, will serve 2 minutes or less if Team B scores.

| Team A | Team B | Player Advantage (pp is power play) |
|---|---|---|
| **4. 5 min. major at 9:38** | **2 min. high sticking at 9:38** | 4 on 4 for first 2 min. Team B pp 5 on 4 last 3 min |

The penalties are not offsetting as the penalties are two different lengths. A player must return to the ice from Team B after 2 minutes to give Team B the player advantage.

| | |
|---|---|
| A goal scored at 8:50 | Both Teams still 4 on 4 so no one returns |
| A goal scored at 7:05 | Team B on pp 5 on 4. Team A player does not return as the player is serving a major |

| Team A | Team B | |
|---|---|---|
| **5. 2 min. holding - #2** | **2 min. high sticking -#5** | #2, #7 offset #5 and #8 |
| **4 min. roughing - #3** | **5 min. fighting - # 15** | Teams play 4 on 4 for 4 min. |
| **2 min. roughing - #7** | **2 min. roughing - #8** | Team A has pp for last min |

A referee can only offset penalties of the same length, so 4 min. and 5 min. penalties cannot be offset and must be fully served. If a goal is scored in the first 4 minutes, no one returns, as Teams are even at 4 on 4 even though one penalty is a major. No reduction of the 2 minute penalties occur either, as the teams are not shorthanded. In the last minute of play, if Team A scores, #15 is not returned to the ice, as the penalty is a major. #2,#5,#7,#8 are returned to the ice at the first whistle after 2 minutes.

| Team A | Team B | Player Advantage (pp is power play) |
|---|---|---|
| **6. 2 min. holding -#2 at 14:35** | **2 min. high sticking -#4 at 13:35** | 14:35 Team B 5 on 4 |
|  |  | 13:35 4 on 4 |
|  | **2 min. roughing - #6 at 13:10** | 13:10 Team A 4 on 3 |
|  |  | 12:35 Team A 5 on 3 |
|  |  | 11:10 5 on 5 |

No offsetting occurs, as penalties occurred at different times. If a goal is scored while a team has the advantage, then the player with the least amount of time is returned. If goal is scored by Team A at 12:06 then #4 returns and Team B is now 1 player short until 11:10.

| | |
|---|---|
| **7. 2 min. roughing #3 at 17:50 (returns 15:50)** | Team A plays 4 on 5 |
| **2 min. high sticking #6 at 16:40 (returns 14:40)** | Team A plays 3 on 5 |
| **2 min. holding #7 at 16:20 (returns 13:50 2 min. after 15:50)** | Team A plays 3 on 5 |

The lowest number of skaters allowed on the ice for any one team is 3. The penalty to #7 must therefore be delayed until the penalty to #3 is completed. If a goal is scored before 15:50 then player #3 is returned to the ice and #7 will start their penalty at that time. Team A will still be playing 3 on 5 until 14:40 when player #6 returns.

**8. 2 min. roughing-#6**          Team B plays 5 on 4
   **(served by #12)**             for 2 min.
   **10 min. misconduct -# 6**

The player #6 will sit out for 12 (10 +2) minutes no matter what happens. Player #12, picked by the coach from the players on the ice, will serve the 2 min. penalty (or less if a goal is scored by Team B). The total penalty is not reduced to #6 for the goal being scored. Player #12 will leave the box early on the goal.

# 25

## What is the Penalty Call Sign Language?

Listed below in pictorial form are the standard calls made by an official during a game. The hand gestures are used by the official to communicate the penalty call to the timekeeper. The use of hand gestures by the referee also allows the fans and coaches to understand the call. Take the time to review the pictures. When a penalty is called people will be able to ask you its meaning, not the other way around.

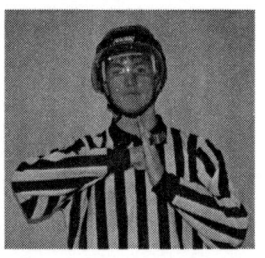

### Boarding

Striking your fist of one hand into the open hand of the other in front of the chest

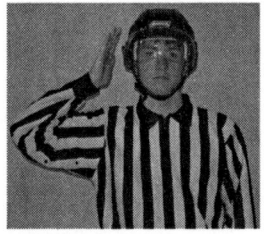

### Checking to the Head

Pat the side of the head with an open hand.

*Hockey For Parents*

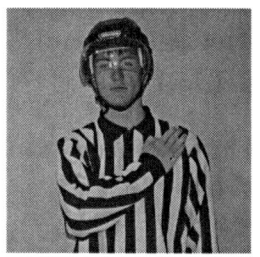

### Bodychecking

Open hand comes up and across the body onto the opposite shoulder.

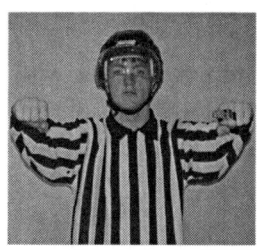

### Cross-Checking

A forward and backward movement of arms with fists clinched simulating holding a hockey stick.

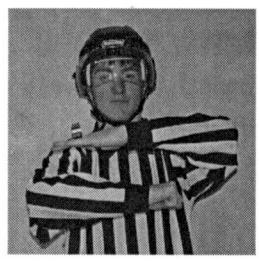

### Butt-Ending

The top arm (with a hand open) crosses over the bottom arm (with a clinched fist).

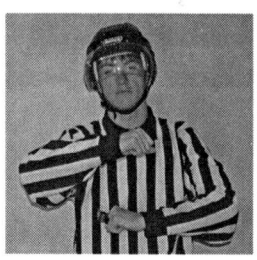

### Charging

Rotate the arms with clinched fists one in front of the other.

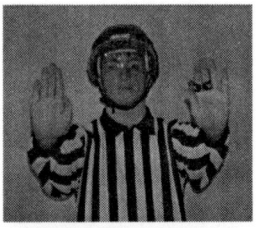

### Checking From Behind

A forward shoving motion with both hands open.

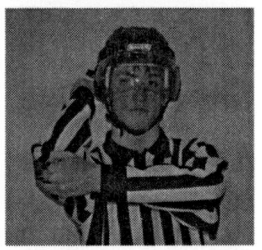

### Elbowing

Grab the elbow with the opposite hand.

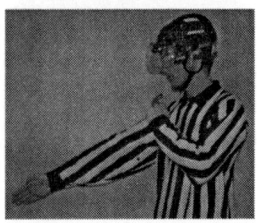

### Goal Scored

Referee points directly toward the ice inside the net area.

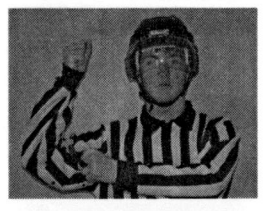

### High Sticking

Simulate holding a hockey stick above the shoulders.

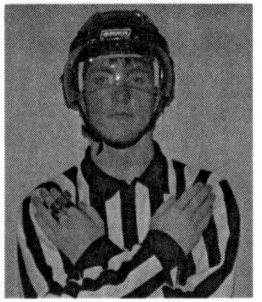

### Interference

Cross your arms in front of your chest with hands open.

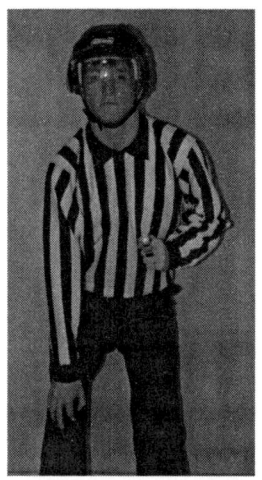

## Kneeing

Pat your knee with your open hand. Keep both feet on the ice.

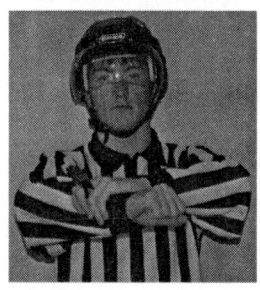

## Holding

Grab your other wrist in front of your body.

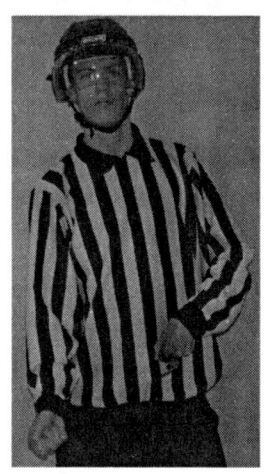

## Holding the Stick

Two stage signal utilizing the holding signal above first. Then second simulate holding a stick.

*Mark James*

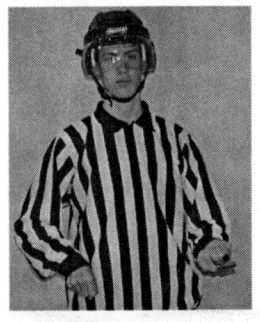

### Hooking

Simulate holding a hockey stick and perform a tugging motion in front of the body.

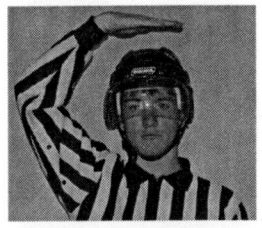

### Match Penalty

Pat the top of the head with an open hand.

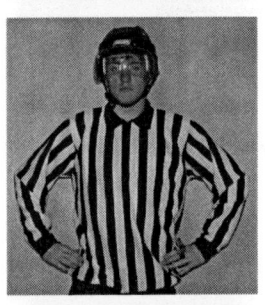

### Misconduct

Put both hands on hips simultaneously.

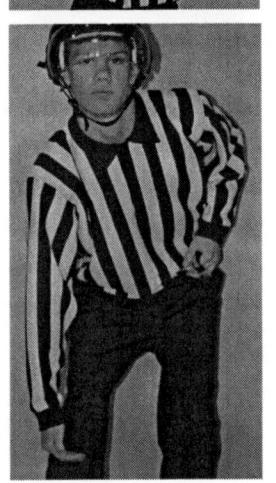

### Tripping

Strike your leg below the knee. Keep both skates on the ice.

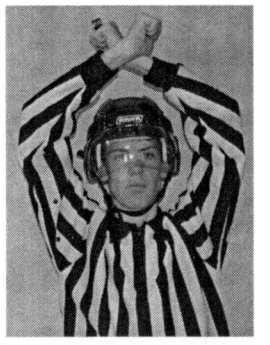

### Penalty Shot

Cross your arms above the head.

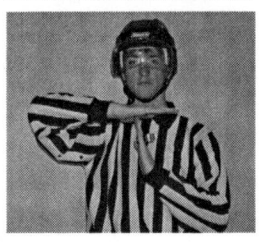

### Unsportmanlike Conduct or Diving

Use both hands to form a "T" in front of the body.

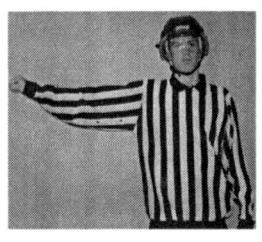

### Roughing

With a clinched fist push your arm out to the side of the body.

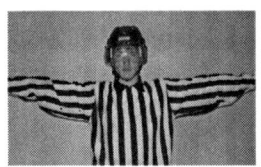

### No Goal/No Icing/ No Offside

Arms extended at shoulder height out wide to the side of the body.

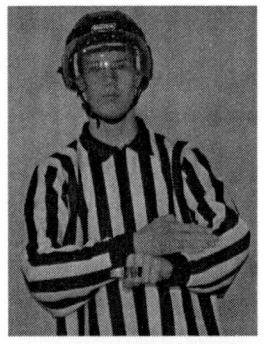

## Slashing

Chop down with an open hand across the other forearm.

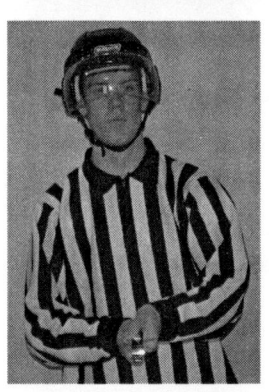

## Spearing

Simulate holding a hockey stick and make a jabbing motion away from the body.

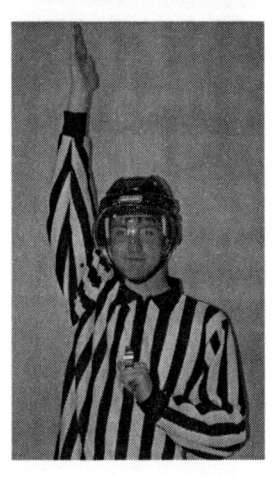

## Icing Call/Delayed Offside Call (Linesman)

Arm is lowered if call is waived off or when the whistle is blown.

## Delayed Penalty Call (Referee)

Arm extended straight above the head until the whistle is blown.

# 26

# THE GAME AND BOOK IS OVER – HOW TO CONTACT US.

I hope that this book has been informative and has earned the right to travel with you in your pocket or purse, to the many arenas you will visit throughout a long hockey season. The size of the book was selected to make it easily portable so that it can always be close at hand.

As coaches or parents, we greatly influence how our children develop and grow, both on and off the ice. It is not an easy job and the pay generally stinks. We take away priceless memories of times spent with our children, and the valued positive comments received from a wide range of contacts such as our team family, other teams' parents and coaches, the rink attendants, the tournament organizers and the referees. These memories will continue to mean more to us than all the trophies and awards that are tucked away in boxes or sit on shelves collecting dust. The true value of hockey is the role it plays in helping us, as parents or coaches, in shaping our young men and women into productive and upstanding adults. We, as parents, must always remember to have fun, and the fun starts with a good understanding of the game. I hope this book has helped with that understanding, and will serve as a strong reference guide. Your children do appreciate your support, even if they forget to tell you as often as they should. The coaches appreciate and need parental support, as they are also hoping to have fun. Never forget that the coaches are devoting a lot of their free time in support of your child. Parents don't miss this opportunity to invest in your child's future while watching the best game in the world. That is the great game we call Hockey!

If you have any questions, feedback or just want to order some more books, I can be reached at markjamesconsulting@rogers.com. The book is available through the Author House website or through Amazon and other retailers. You can find the book on Google by typing in Hockey for Parents.

PLAY SMART, PLAY HARD, PLAY SAFE
AND PLAY FOR THE LOVE OF THE GAME

# 27
## Glossary

**Angling** – this is a skating direction taken by a player to force an opposing player to move in a desired direction. Angling, if done correctly, does not allow an opposing player to reverse direction or avoid pressure from the attacking player.

**Back-check** – Players without the puck skating towards their own end to assist defensively.

**Body Check** – this term is used for a player using their body to make contact with an opposing player's body in an attempt to free the puck from the puck carrier.

**The Box** – a defensive zone coverage position in which 4 players take a position that forms a box shape with players at the 4 corners. The goal of the box is to keep the offensive players with the puck outside of the box.

**Breakout** – A team in control of the puck in their own zone attempting to leave their zone by passing or carrying the puck. A controlled breakout is a term used when the defenseman generally stops behind the net, and waits for their players to get into position before starting the break out.

**Control** – keeping a player away from your goal without committing to make a hit.

**Deflection** – when a player, generally in front of the opposition net, uses their stick or body to change the direction of the puck. If this player is the last to touch the puck before a goal is scored, this player will be credited with the goal.

**Dump In** – releasing the puck to the opposition in their end in an effort to move the puck further away from our goal. Generally done to avoid the trap, or execute a player change.

**Face-off** – after each whistle the start of play occurs with a face-off at one of the red dots on the ice (there are eight). All players from one team must be on one side of the dot closest to their end and all players from the other team must be on the other side of the dot closer to their end.

**Fore-check** – One team applying pressure in the offensive zone to recover the puck.

**The Gap** – this is the area of ice any where on the ice between an offensive player and the defensive player in coverage.

**Go wide** – a player moving outside the opposition defenseman close to the boards. Players should "go wide" to create space and use the entire ice surface.

**Hash Marks**- The two lines on either side of the circles located inside the blue line. The purpose of these two lines is to separate the player's body and their sticks from touching each other prior to a face-off. Encroachment by stick or body prior to the puck being dropped should result in the center of the encroaching player being removed from the face-off.

**Icing** – shooting the puck down the ice at even player strength from your side of center ice to over the red line that extends from the goal line.

**Lanes** – these are generally straight line openings in the defense which would allow a pass or puck carrier to move unimpeded.

**Misconduct Penalty** – generally the penalty is called as a result of player's improper behaviour, either verbal or physical, after or during the play.

**Gross Misconduct Penalty** – generally attached to a serious misconduct penalty (abuse of an official) or applied to a normal penalty call that was determined by the referee to have caused serious injury, or there was intent to cause serious injury. A Gross Misconduct generally results in additional game suspensions. See chapter 28.

**On the Fly** – this term is used when the clock is running down and a team makes a change, pulls a goalie etc. as opposed to after the whistle is blown.

**Offsetting** – when penalties of equal value are served, but no team plays short handed.

**Pass** – a player moving the puck from their stick to a teammate's stick.

**Power Play** – any time one team has more skaters on the ice than the other team, due to penalties.

**Penalty Kill** – due to penalties one team has fewer skaters on the ice. This team is allowed to ice the puck.

**Shot** – any attempt to score on the net by an offensive player. A shot on goal, which is preferred, hits the net. If you are asked to do statistics for the team, then only count the shots that hit the goal and would have gone in the net if the goalie was not there. Hitting the post or crossbar is not a shot on goal, as the puck would not go into the net, with or without the goalie.

**Space** – open area of the ice where no player is standing. The bigger the space the more time afforded the player to make the correct decision.

**Stick handling or Carrying the Puck** – a player controlling the puck with their stick as they move on the ice.

**Trap** – a defensive strategy of having forwards hang back in the neutral area to clog up the lanes and avoid odd man rushes for the opposition. This is generally used to protect a lead.

**Our Zone (Defensive Zone)** – the area of ice from inside our blue-line to the boards behind our goal.

**Their Zone (Offensive Zone)** – the area of ice from the opponent's blue-line to the boards behind their net.

**Neutral Zone** – the area between the blue lines where the player's benches and the penalty/timekeeper box is located.

# 28

## Penalty Suspensions

Pages have been added so that you can obtain from your hockey association a list of suspensions detailed by the codes put on a game sheet. You could then attach them to these pages. Every association has different rules and length of suspension for each infraction so one list cannot be printed. The question asked after every game in which a player is removed from the game for a serious penalty is "How long will that suspension be?" Once you have added the suspension list you can turn to these pages and offer the answer.

LaVergne, TN USA
29 October 2009
162350LV00001B/2/P